W. W. Rittmann · S. M. Perren

Cortical Bone Healing after Internal Fixation and Infection

Biomechanics and Biology

With the Collaboration of
M. Allgöwer · F. H. Kayser · J. Brennwald

With 65 Partly Coloured Figures
(154 Separate Illustrations)

Springer-Verlag
Berlin Heidelberg New York 1974

PD. Dr. med. W. W. RITTMANN, Department of Surgery of the University of Basel, Kantonsspital, CH-4004 Basel

PD. Dr. med. S. M. PERREN, Director of the Laboratory for Experimental Surgery, Swiss Research Institut, CH-7270 Davos

ISBN-13:978-3-642-65979-9 e-ISBN-13:978-3-642-65977-5
DOI: 10.1007/978-3-642-65977-5

Library of Congress Cataloging in Publication Data. RITTMANN, W. W., 1938– Cortical bone healing after internal fixation and infection. Translation of Corticale Knochenheilung nach Osteosynthese und Infektion. Bibliography: p. 1. Bone-grafting. 2. Bone regeneration. 3. Surgery-Complications and sequelae. I. PERREN STEPHAN, M., 1932– joint author. II. Title. [DNLM: 1. Fracture fixation, Internal. 2. Wound healing WE180 R615c] RD123.R5713 616.7'1 74-16465

Foreword

The danger of infection remains the most serious drawback to internal fixation. Prevention, using all available prophylactic measures should be the central feature in every surgical department. Though the infection rate may remain below the acceptable level of 2%, the infected patient derives little comfort from the large number of excellent results in other people. We must discover the best way to offer these patients a favourable prognosis. This should not be based on intuition but on clear proven guiding principles.

Planning the treatment for a patient whose internal fixation has become septic must decide between steps which may have advantages or disadvantages. The disadvantage of the presence of a foreign body must be weighed against the advantage of rigidity. The authors have taken up this challenge by planned animal experiments to study the healing of internally fixed fractures which have been infected with staphylococci. They have shown that under stable conditions, even massive infection did not destroy the healing process in cortical bone. Even under these circumstances fracture union, in the form of primary bone healing, can occur even if with less regularity than in uninfected internal fixation.

It would perhaps not be right to publish the overall results in the form of a monograph, where it not of great practical interest for the surgeon to be able to follow the planned steps in the experiment and the evaluation of the results. In this study the surgeon will find valuable suggestions about achieving rigidity in these fractures as well as on the treatment of his hopefully few infected cases. For many, moreover, it will be a real pleasure to follow step by step fundamental research directly related to patient care.

M. Allgoewer

Foreword

Contents

1. Introduction and Purpose of the Experiment 1

2. Material and Methods 4
2.1. Group Division 4
2.2. Material 4
2.2.1. Experimental Animals 4
2.2.2. Bacteria 4
2.2.3. Implants 4
2.3. Methods 7
2.3.1. Anaesthesia and Operative Procedure 7
2.3.2. Measurement of Interfragmentary Compression 10
2.3.3. Measurement of Torque of the Screws 12
2.3.4. Measurement of Weight Bearing 13
2.3.5. Infection and Control of Infectious Process 13
2.3.6. Radiologic Examination 16
2.3.6.1. Plain Film X-Rays 16
2.3.6.2. Microangiography 16
2.3.6.3. Microradiography 16
2.3.7. Polychrome Sequential Labelling and Histological Preparation 16
2.4. Summary of the Experimental Protocol 18

3. Results 19
3.1. General Aspects 19
3.2. Local Infection 20
3.3. Interfragmentary Compression 26
3.4. Torque of the Screws 35
3.5. Loading Force 36
3.6. X-Rays: Plain Films 40
3.7. Histological Examination 49

4. Discussion 63

5. Summary and Conclusions 70

Acknowledgments 71

Literature 72

Subject Index 75

1. Introduction and Purpose of the Experiment

"The risk of infection remains the crucial issue of internal fixation" (ALLGOEWER, 1971) [3]. The surgical exposure of the fracture zone, necrosis of soft tissue and bone (produced by trauma and operation), as well as foreign body reactions to the implants enhance local growth and spread of infection. In spite of infection a fracture can heal under favourable biomechanical conditions as observed in clinical experience. Thus, the changes in the biomechanical response of the bone to a local infection are of primary interest.

The *frequency* of bone infections after operative management as reported in the literature varies from 0.54 to 6.6% for closed fractures [41, 110, 91, 3] and from 3.7 to 15% for compound fractures [41, 75, 95, 105, 74].

The *significance* of bone infections becomes evident from the rate of amputation. Two thirds of the amputations following lower leg fractures are a consequence of infection, as reported by HICKS [43] in 1964[1]. In the total material of compound and closed fractures presented by HICKS [41] the amputation rate was 0.4%. KUNER *et al.* [63] reported a 6% amputation rate when related to bone infections. After predominantly conservative management of fractures ELLIS [24] reported 2.8%, HOLDERMANN [52] 9%, DEHNE *et al.* [19] 0% and SCOTT [101] 0.8% amputations.

The clinical and therapeutic considerations of bone infection are treated extensively in four recent textbooks (HIERHOLZER *et al.* [50], 1970; POPKIROV [86], 1971; WALDVOGEL *et al.* [107], 1971; BURRI [14], 1974).

The *bacteria* most frequently implicated in post-traumatic osteitis as cited by all recent statistics [38, 11, 48, 68, 76, 63, 86] continues to be *staphylococcus aureus*. This organism can be found in 54–93% of the infections. In about 50% of the cases it is associated with other bacteria [38, 25, 63]. Very often, staphylococci alone are found at the onset of the disease [11, 50] while later in the course a super- or reinfection [102], predominantly with *proteus sp.*, *E. coli*, *pseudomonas sp.*, streptococci and *staphylococcus epidermidis* occurs. As a consequence of such contamination, FEISCHL [25] believes that the healing process is impaired, and reports a prolongation of the average hospital stay in his patients from 3.8 to 6.7 months.

The *radiologic* changes are characterised by spotty sites of diminished bone density appearing in the third week [26] and showing a tendency to become confluent later. In addition, subperiosteal bony apposition occurs during the same period [33], and, after the fourth week, so-called "sclerosis" of the fracture ends appears [107]. In many cases sequestra can be recognised on the basis of their relative opacity on X-ray. They do not however, appear before 2 months, and occasionally not before one year [45]. CHARKES *et al.* [15] attribute the delay in appearance of the first radiologic signs to the fact that a 30–50% loss of calcium compounds must occur before radiologic changes become evident. The X-ray manifestations found in experimental osteitis of the rabbit infected with staphylococci are reported by NORDEN [80] to be similar to those radiologic manifestations found in

[1] It is of historical interest that BILLROTH [9] amputated in 40% of his compound fractures between 1860 and 1867 while LISTER [69] in 1867 lost 1 out of 13 extremities treated for compound fractures.

humans. But studies correlating the radiologic changes with the histological alterations are still lacking.

Some of the *histological* manifestations of bone infections have been described by LENNERT [65], HICKS [45], HIERHOLZER *et al.* [50], POPKIROV [86] and WALDVOGEL *et al.* [107][2]. The following changes were found to be typical: a central necrosis with fibrin deposits and massive polynuclear infiltration; a well vascularised granulation tissue with lymphocytes and plasma cells appears and surrounds the area of central necrosis; then follows scar tissue and finally sclerotic bone. Dead bone is thought to be caused by vessel thrombosis supposedly due to spreading of the infection along the Haversian and Volkmann's canals. This necrotic bone is reported to be free from osteocytes, connective tissue and bone marrow cells. On occasion new bone deposition by osteoblasts is found on necrotic trabeculae. The opinion that the whole area is underperfused is shared by many additional authors [21, 11, 71, 67]. A secondary revascularisation of formerly dead bone seems to be possible [109]. In addition, formation of a cloudy callus is characteristic for the disease. It remains to be shown how the different processes are interrelated and what the time sequence of their appearance is.

LANE [64] was the first surgeon to recognise the infectious origin of the tissue reactions following plating. *Therapy* has since become more specific but bone infection remains exceptionally refractory to treatment, "a disease which never heals up" [47, 14]. Some specific aspects of medical therapy have recently gained additional significance: the effectiveness of the local application of antibiotics [109, 21, 39, 20, 82]; systemic chemoprophylaxis [104, 18, 57, 95, 27, 32, 86], determination of antibiotic tissue levels [46, 97, 67, 81], as well as local tissue toxicity [60]. The surgical management of the disease offers no uniform solution. Some authors [92, 96, 108] emphasise only the foreign body effect of the implants and recommend, without compromise, removal of all metal as soon as an infection is manifest. Or, they may accept only "that one or two screws holding the fracture well may be left until union occurs". The danger of this approach is the development of an infected pseudarthrosis. Other authors [35, 20, 45, 71, 82, 3] place emphasis on the stabilising function of the implants and recommend leaving implants which still offer stability in place in the infected area until bony union of the fragments is secured. These latter authors accept a prolonged period of soft tissue infection in return for the advantage of bone healing. There is, however, good agreement with the concept that implants which no longer offer stability must be removed. However there is no concensus of opinion regarding which implant would be preferred in restabilising such fractures. Some authors [38, 77] prefer the intramedullary rod, others utilise plates and still others prefer external fixation devices (first developed by KEY [61, 16] and recently popularised again [78, 3]). When one is faced with an infection, the decision as to whether or not metal should be left in, or put in and of which type and quantity should be based on the anticipated reaction of the infectious disease and bone healing to the metal implanted.

It would be of interest to examine the role of *biomechanical* factors in the healing process of the infected fractures. How long will stability last in the presence of local infection? Will infection as such produce bone resorption and thereby loss of *interfragmentary compression*, that factor (first clinically introduced by DANIS [17] in 1947) which has been shown to be of extraordinary importance in primary bone healing. Many authors have demonstrated its importance in their clinical experience [4, 79, 2]. Is primary bone healing at all possible under conditions of infection? Of what significance is it finally, whether an infected fracture heals by first or second intention? Is it correct, as HICKS [44] says, that "the details of fracture healing, whether by first intention or otherwise, were of secondary importance"?

Little *experimental work* has been done in the field of osteitis. Of historical interest are the experiments of HUNTER [54], who early in the 19th century tested the effectiveness of different

[2] Often no clear distinction is made between haematogenous and posttraumatic osteitis.

surgical procedures as well as the work of KOCHER [62] (1878) and LEXER [66] (1924), who studied an experimental model for creating bone infection. Recent work has dealt predominantly with factors of the pathogenesis [98, 34, 53, 23, 11, 36], or with treatment by means of bone grafts [8], as well as pharmacological aspects [81] of bone infection. Little has been done to study the healing pattern of infected fractures [70]. Biomechanical factors under conditions of bone infection have, to our knowledge, not been studied, except for the unpublished experiments done by B. FRIEDRICH (personal communication *).

It is the *purpose* of the present experiments to study cortical bone healing after internal fixation in the face of local infection, with special emphasis placed on the changes occurring with interfragmentary compression. In addition, the changes on X-ray examination available to the clinician will be correlated with additional information obtained from histology, bacteriology and mechanics of the experiment.

---

* Meanwhile published: FRIEDRICH, B.: Die Bedeutung der biomechanischen Stabilität in der Ätiologie der posttraumatischen Osteomyelitis; Würzburg: Habilitationsschrift (1973).

2. Material and Methods

We examined cortical bone healing in the presence of a staphylococcal infection in three groups, which differed from each other by the type of plate fixation utilised.

2.1. Group Division

In Fig. 1 the different groups are listed. The methods of internal fixation applied are chosen to allow immediate and unrestricted weight bearing by the use of relatively heavy implants.

— Internal fixation with two small plates producing compression at the osteotomy planes. This group of 9 animals will be called "compression with two gauge plates".

— Internal fixation by the use of one broad plate applying compression on the fracture planes (group "compression with one plate"). In this group of 7 animals the clinical procedure of a compression-osteosynthesis utilising only one plate on the tibia shaft was simulated. However, because of the expected immediate full weight bearing in the animal, a broad plate, larger than would ordinarily be used in relation to the tibia was applied.

— Internal fixation by the use of a "flexible" broad plate without applying interfragmentary compression (group "no compression with one plate"). In this group of 9 animals a certain instability was aimed at by reduction of the plate diameter in the midportion and by avoiding interfragmentary compression. The gap between the fracture ends was standardised at 100 µm.

In order to evaluate the changes in interfragmentary compression of an infected plate fixation *in vivo,* implants equipped with strain gauge elements (so-called "gauge plates") were used in one group of animals (group "compression with two gauge plates"). With these plates long term pressure recordings throughout the healing period could be registered.

2.2. Material

2.2.1. Experimental Animals

Mountain sheep, 2–3 years old, of both sexes (males castrated) were used as experimental animals. They were kept in individual boxes of a stable and given water and hay *ad libitum.*

2.2.2. Bacteria

The infection was instituted with *staphylococcus aureus* of the phage type 47/53/54/75, isolated from a human staphylococcal infection. The lyophilised organisms were supplied by F. H. Kayser from the Institute for Medical Microbiology, University of Zürich, Switzerland. Virulence was enhanced by blood agar plate and mice passages (see p. 14, 15).

2.2.3. Implants

Plates and screws made of a titanium-oxygen alloy were used. The composition and physical properties are summarised in Table 1. Corrosion resistance of titanium in body fluids is excellent

GROUP	IMPLANT	OSTEOTOMY	QUESTION
"Compres-sion with two gauge plates"	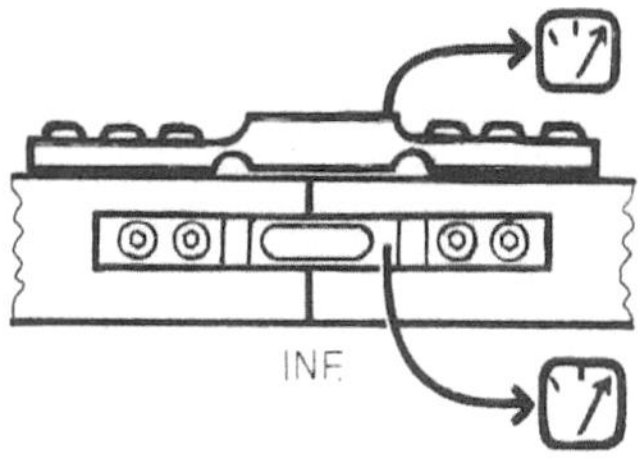	contact stability	Healing course under conditions of rigid internal fixation by the use of compression. Measurement of interfragmentary compression changes.
"Compres-sion with one plate"	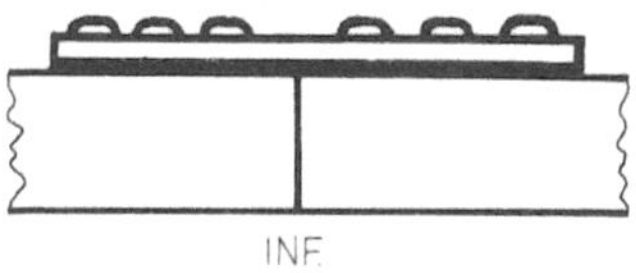	contact stability	Healing course under stable conditions using one broad plate and applying interfragmentary compression.
"No com-pression with one plate"	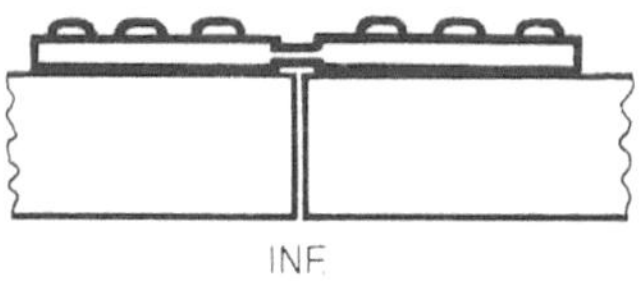	gap (100 µm) moderate instabil-ity	Healing course under conditions of moderate instability due to the lack of interfragmentary compression and fixation with a "flexible" plate.

Fig. 1. Synopsis of the three experimental groups: Experimental model, implants used and question to be studied in the respective experimental group

[51, 103]. The tissue tolerance was tested by BECHTOL *et al.* [7] and was found to be quite satisfactory. Due to the low stiffness of titanium the functional stresses in the plated bone segment are reduced less and only partial stress protection results underneath the plate, as shown by BRENNWALD *et al.* [12]. The design of the plates corresponds to the dynamic compression plate (DCP) of the ASIF [3], formerly described in detail by PERREN *et al.* [84].

The specific geometry of the screw holes (Fig. 2) causes traction on the plate and thereby axial compression on the bone when the screws are driven home (Fig. 3).

By modification of this dynamic compression plate the special conditions for the three experimental groups were provided.

[3] Association for the study of internal fixation.

Table 1. Chemical analysis and mechanical properties of the plate material used (titanium): The implants were made of a so-called "non-alloyed" titanium. The composition is given in percentage by weight. The mechanical properties listed relate to the condition of the metal after the manufacturing process and after cold deformation. The metal corresponds to the quality standards of the Swiss Association for standardisation (SNV Nr. 056507)

Chemical analysis	
Titanium	99.35% min.
Oxygen	0.50% max.
Iron	0.30% max.
Carbon	0.10% max.
Hydrogen	0.015% max.
Mechanical properties	
Tensile strength	≧ 700 N/mm²
Tensile elongation to failure (50 mm length of probe)	≧ 18%
Bending angle before crack (inner diameter of curvature = probe thickness)	≧ 60°
Modulus of elasticity	1.1×10^5 N/mm²

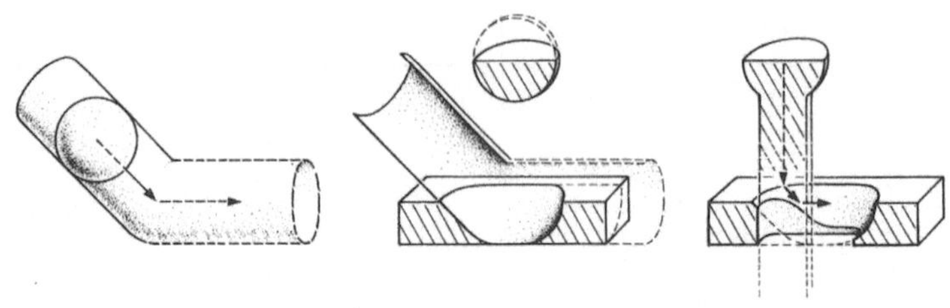

Fig. 2. The screw hole of the dynamic compression plate (DCP[4]): The geometry of the screw hole causes axial compression in the bone when the spherical screw head glides down the sloped plane. a. "Ball-glide-principle": a ball is guided in a sloped cylinder (load track) and horizontal cylinder (glide plane). b. The screw head is spherically formed. The screw hole is composed of two cylindrical segments. c. Correlation between screw and screw hole on longitudinal section. (From PERREN *et al.* [84])

Gauge Plate. A measuring chamber was placed between the two inner holes of a small dynamic compression plate of the ASIF, type 423. This compartment contains strain gauge elements for registration of axial forces (see p. 10).

Dynamic Compression Plate, Type 425. A broad ASIF-plate, type 425, was used without change in design in the group "compression with one plate".

Flexible Plate. The midportion of a broad dynamic compression plate of the ASIF, type 425, was rendered more flexible by reduction of its thickness from 5 to 3 mm between the inner two holes. The calculated moment of inertia equalled 36.0 mm^4.

The screws used in the plates were of the type 414, ASIF. The screw heads were spherical to fit the geometrical design of the screw holes.

The operative procedures were performed using the ASIF instruments and adapting the technique described in the ASIF manual for internal fixation [79].

[4] Dynamic compression plate of the ASIF.

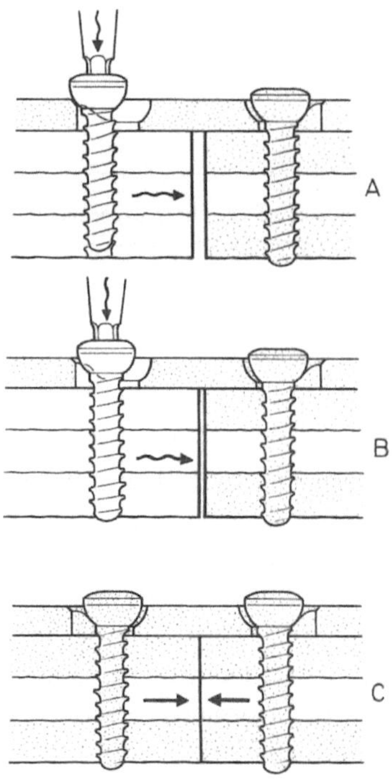

Fig. 3. Axial compression on bone by the use of a dynamic compression plate: The sloped plane in the holes makes it possible to exert axial compression on the osteotomy plane without the use of an external compression device. With a first screw the implant is fixed to one main fragment. Driving the second screw home (A to C) along the sloped plane of the screw hole moves the second main fragment (⇝) towards the osteotomy plane. After complete adaptation, an axial force (→) causes traction on the plate and compression on the osteotomy

2.3. Methods

2.3.1. Anaesthesia and Operative Procedure

Following a 48 hour period of fasting, the animals received Atropine i.m. 0.4 mg/kg body weight[5]. A central venous catheter of 1.5 mm diameter was inserted percutaneously into the external jugular vein and 500 ml of D5W were begun. Anaesthesia was initiated with sodium penthobarbital (Nembutal). A standard dose of 10 mg/kg body weight was varied individually until the lid reflexes and the reflexes of swallowing had just disappeared and the muscles of mastication became relaxed. Intubation was then performed using a tracheal tube of 10 mm diameter. Narcosis was performed using a Fluothane-oxygen mixture in a semiclosed system (2–3 liters/min flow). Fluothane concentrations varied between 1–2.5 volume %. An increase in respiratory rate or return of spontaneous muscular activity prompted an increase in the dosage. The gastric contents were drained using a tube of 20 mm diameter in order to avoid respiratory impairment due to air accumulation in the different stomachs, a result of fermentation at a time when the animal was incapable of regurgitation.

The operative procedure was performed under sterile conditions after placing the animal in a right lateral decubitus position. The right leg was shaved, degreased with ether, disinfected with Desogen, and covered by means of Vi-Drape spray and plastic foil drape. Through a medio-posterior incision equalling the length of the implant, the right tibia was exposed, preserving the periosteum. The osteotomy was performed in the midshaft area using an oscillating saw with a blade of 100 μm thickness. Thermal damage to the bone was minimised by constant irrigation with a cooled Ringer's lactate solution. The stabilisation of the osteotomy was performed using the ASIF dynamic compression plates (see p. 5). While the screws were driven home the torque of each screw was measured (see p. 12).

[5] This is a much higher dose of Atropine than that used in human anaesthesia.

At termination of the procedure a negative pressure drainage was used for 24–48 hours. The skin was sutured with one layer of 4-0 Dermalon sutures using intracutaneous, interrupted stitches. The wound was then protected by Nobecutan spray and no dressing was applied. After extubation and awakening from the anaesthesia, the animal was brought into the stable, where it was allowed to bear its full weight immediately without additional external splints.

The detailed procedure of internal fixation will be described for the three different groups:

Group *"compression with two gauge plates"*. In nine sheep a 6-hole DCP plate was affixed to the medial side of the tibia, as well as a 4-hole DCP plate which was placed posteriorly. Both implants were equipped with strain gauge compartments (see p. 6). Axial compression on the osteotomy was exerted by specific and controlled eccentric placement of the screws in the screw holes.

The procedures utilised in this group were performed in the following steps:

- Prior to the osteotomy the location of the two plates was planned. This was determined by placing them at levels which differed from each other by one half the distance between two holes of the plates when measured longitudinally.
- Both plates were adapted to the bone surface by bending, utilising two Steinemann pins passed through the screw holes as bending devices.
- The two inner holes of both plates were then drilled, one by the use of the neutral drill guide in the centre of the screw hole (centrically) and one using the load guide for drilling 1.0 mm eccentrically.
- The drill holes were tapped.
- Therafter the osteotomy was performed.
- The implants were reattached, driving home the inner two screws into the tapped drill holes. As a consequence of the eccentric position of the screws a static axial compression could be exerted on the osteotomy planes and the osteotomy gap disappeared macroscopically (Fig. 4).

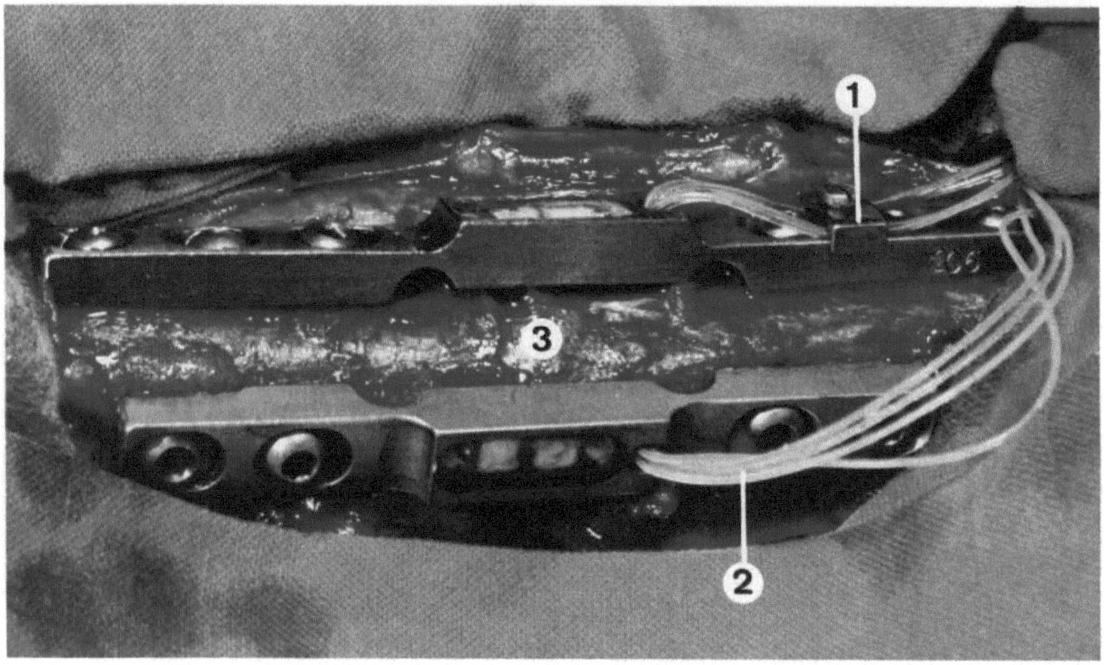

Fig. 4. Intraoperative view in group "compression with two gauge plates": A 6-hole gauge plate on the medial, a 4-hole gauge plate on the posterior surface of the tibia. The electrical wires of the 6-hole plate are attached to the plate using a metal clip (1). The wires of the 4-hole plate (2) are not yet fixed to the implant. In between the two strain gauge chambers the transverse osteotomy (3) is barely visible. The periosteum was preserved intact

— All other screws were inserted centrically within the screw holes, which resulted in a slight additional axial compression.

The wire connection coming from the strain gauge chamber was fixed against the plate by means of a metal clip to avoid a rupture at the region near the chamber. By use of a sharp pointed guide, the wires were conducted subcutaneously to the area of the greater femoral trochanter, where they were passed through the skin and were preserved in a small pocket sutured to the skin externally.

Group *"compression with one plate":* In seven sheep a broad 6-hole DCP plate was used to obtain a rigid internal fixation. Compression was achieved by specific placement of the screws in the screw holes.

The internal fixation procedure included the following steps:

— The 6-hole DCP plate was adapted to the medial surface of the tibia by bending, so that a space of approx. 2 mm remained between the undersurface of the midportion of the plate and the adjacent bone cortex where the osteotomy was planned. This should result in so-called "prebending" [61] (Fig. 5) adding axial compression to the osteotomy plane in the bone cortex opposite the plate.

— The first of the two inner holes was placed centrically in neutral position within the screw hole of the plate. The other was placed eccentrically using the load guide. Both holes were then drilled and tapped.

— An osteotomy was performed after the drilling and tapping of the holes.

— Afterwards, with insertion of the two inner screws, there resulted an axial compression

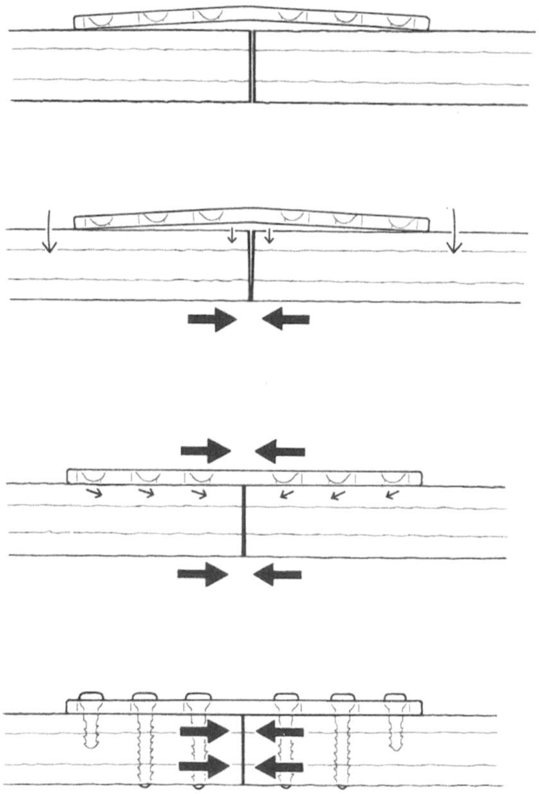

◁ Fig. 5. Principle of "prebending" of the plate: By driving home eccentrically placed screws through a "pre-loaded" plate, axial compression is exerted on the entire osteotomy plane. In this manner the gap between the main fragments closes also on the cortex opposite to the plate. This technique was used in the group "compression with one plate"

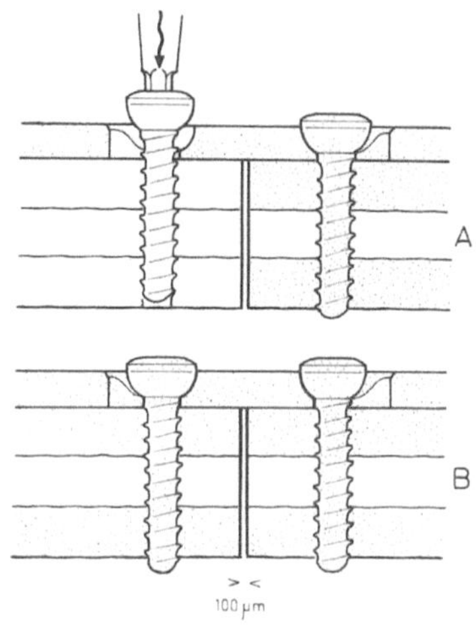

Fig. 7. Maintainance of a gap between the fragment ends: The screws are placed at the inner end of the sloped cylinder segment of the screw holes in the plate (A), which avoids closure of the 100 µm wide gap, when they are driven home (B)

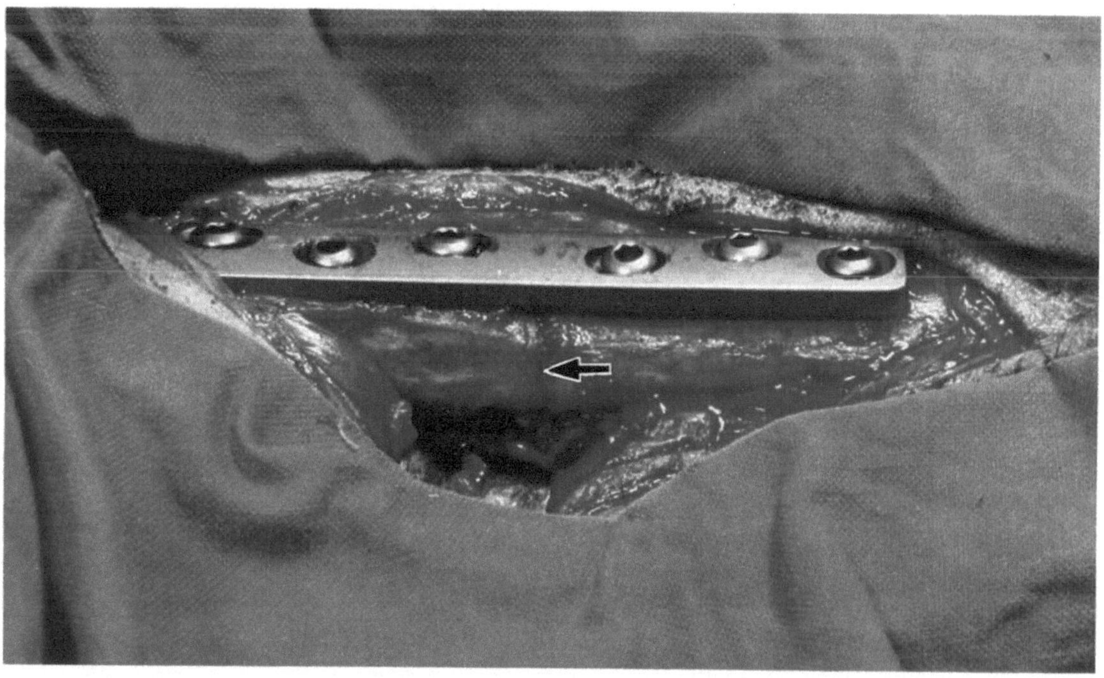

Fig. 6. Intraoperative view in group "compression with one plate": The plate is located on the medial side of the tibia. Prebending of the plate and eccentric location of the screws within the screw holes leads to axial compression of the entire osteotomy plane and closes the gap between the main fragments (←) almost completely

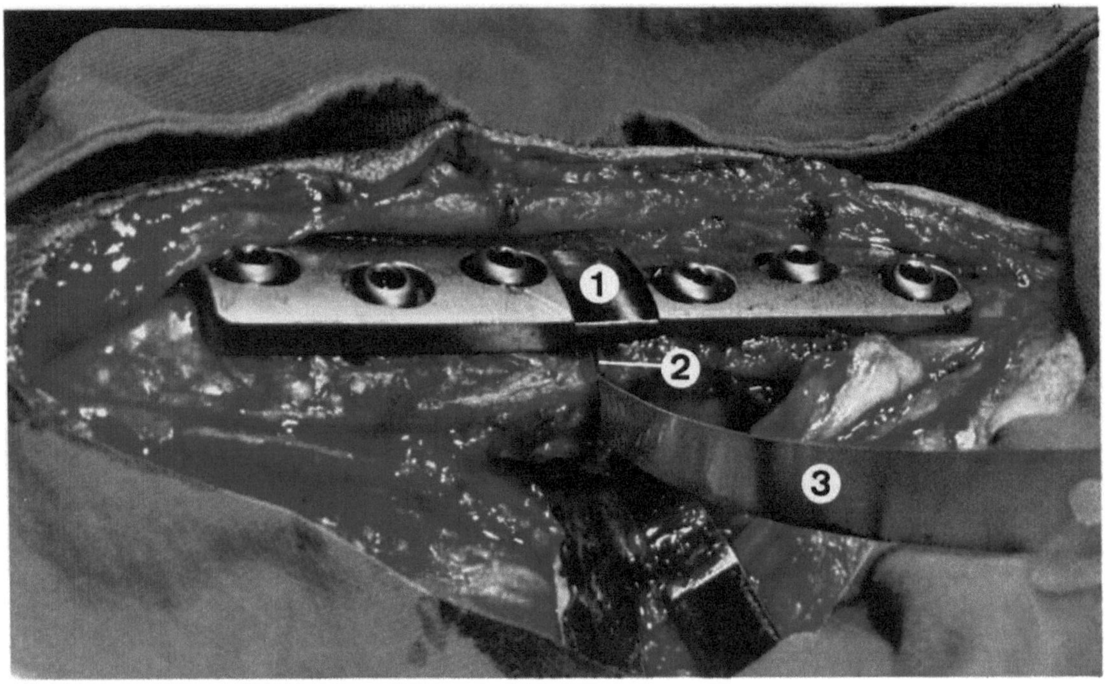

Fig. 8. Intraoperative view in group "no compression with one plate": The 6-hole DCP is placed on the medial site of the tibia. The midsegment of the plate showing the reduction in cross section (1) lies directly over the easily recognisable osteotomy (2). A metal guide plate (3) of 100 µm thickness is inserted temporarily in between the two main fragments for standardisation of the gap size

of the entire osteotomy plane as a consequence of the eccentric screw position and of the "prebending" of the plate.
- All other screws were placed centrically within the screw holes which resulted in slight additional axial compression (Fig. 6).

Group *"no compression with one plate":* In nine sheep a moderately unstable bridging of the osteotomy was attempted by the use of a single plate with a reduced cross section in the midportion of the plate. By special arrangement of the screws within the screw holes the entire osteotomy gap was held apart.

The internal fixation procedure was performed as here described:
- Prior to performing the osteotomy the broad 6-hole DCP plate was adapted to the medial bone surface very precisely.
- One of the two inner screws was again placed centrically within the screw hole, while atypically, the second one lay eccentric near the *inner* border of the screw hole. This prevented the gliding action of the plate and maintained a "zero-load" situation on the bone.
- The osteotomy was then performed.
- A metal guide plate of 100 µm thickness was inserted between the two fragment ends to maintain the gap open, while the inner two screws were driven home (Figs. 7 and 8).
- After insertion of the remaining screws in neutral position, the tightly held metal plate between the fragments could be removed leaving a standardised distance of 100 µm between the fragment ends.

2.3.2. Measurement of Interfragmentary Compression

Longitudinal compression on the osteotomy planes could be measured in the sheep of group "compression with two gauge plates" using strain gauge elements placed into the chamber of the plate. This method is based on the fact that forces acting

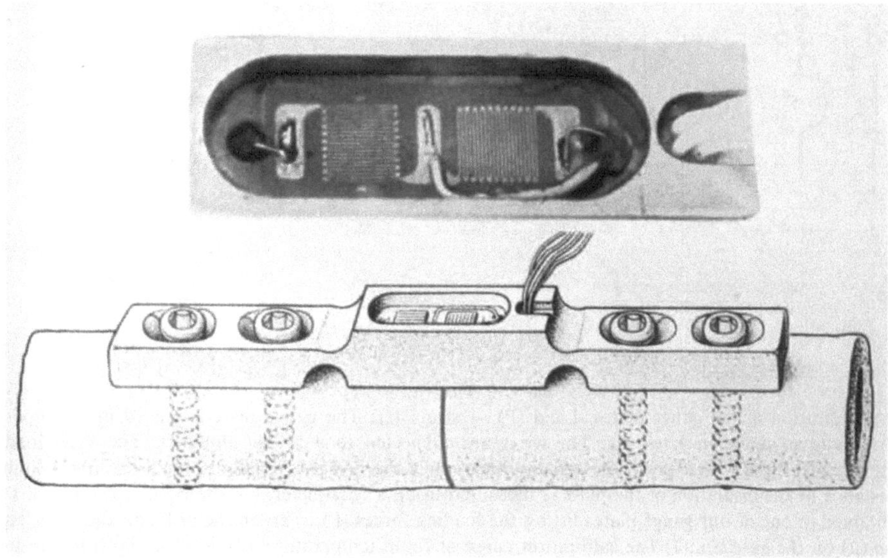

Fig. 9. Schematic drawing of the gauge plate and photographic view of the strain gauge chamber in detail: The dynamic compression plate is modified by insertion of a chamber between the inner two screw holes which contains strain gauge elements. Four wires connect the chamber of the implant with the measuring devices outside the animal. The segment between strain gauge chamber and the remaining part of the plate is reduced in diameter, resembling so-called "plastic joints". These junctions prevent plastic deformations by bending and torsion stresses in the segment carrying the gauge chamber. Above: Photographic insert showing the gauge chamber. The arrangement of the strain gauge elements along the longitudinal and transverse axes of the plate is clearly recognisable

in the longitudinal axis of the plate lead to changes in the length of the plate (strain) [83]. These strains are proportional to the forces applied and cause respective changes in the electrical resistance of the contained strain gauge elements. Such changes in resistance cause a disturbance of the electrical equilibrium of the Wheatstone bridge portion of the strain gauge elements and originate thereby force-dependent potentials. The implanted plates are connected to phase-sensitive carrier frequency amplifiers outside the animal by wire connection.

The strain gauge elements were located in a chamber between the two inner screw holes (Fig. 9). By appropriate arrangement of the gauge elements only longitudinal forces were registered. Bending forces could affect only minimally the elastic deformation of the metal support underneath the strain gauge elements, since it was placed near the neutral axis. The remaining effect of the bending forces was mostly compensated electrically (Wheatstone bridge). Plastic deformation by bending and torsion stresses could be eliminated by "plastic joints" on both sides of the gauge chamber connecting the measuring devices from the remaining plate. Effects from temperature changes finally were compensated by the appropriate arrangement of the strain gauge elements. As a result, only variations in *longitudinal* forces could cause alterations in the electrical resistance of the strain gauge elements.

A direct proportional relation thus existed between the transmitted signal from the strain gauge elements and the magnitude of longitudinal stress. This linear relationship was tested prior to implantation as well as after explantation at room temperature and at 37° C. For this purpose, the plate was mounted in a test rig and loaded in the axial direction by use of a Jack-screw (Fig. 10). By balancing the bridge amplifier the changes in resistance of the strain gauge elements could be correlated with the longitudinal traction applied.

Since defects of the insulation of wires or chamber can simulate alterations in strain gauge

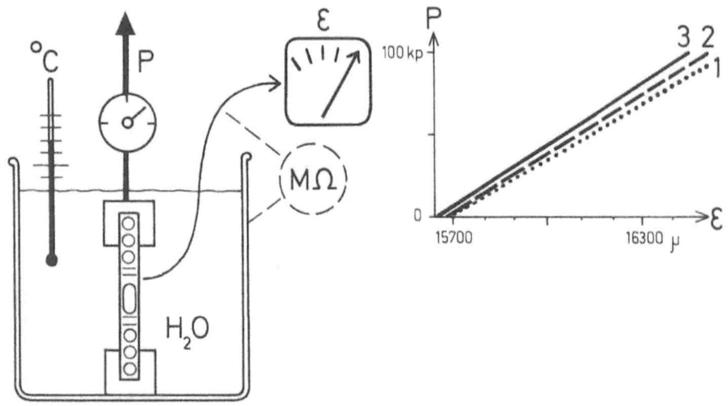

Fig. 10. Calibration of the gauge plates. Load (P) → strain (ε): The gauge plate is placed in a temperature controlled water bath and mounted in a test rig. The wires are connected to a bridge amplifier. The axial load (P) applied by Jack-screw is measured with a precision dynamometer while the bridge amplifier permits reading of indicated strain (ε). The resistance of the insulation of the plate is measured using a MΩ-meter. On the right: Example of a load-strain diagram obtained in one of our gauge plates listing the loading forces (P) in kp on the ordinate and the changes in strain (ε) in µm/m (µ) on the abscissa. (1) The calibration curve at room temperature, (2) at 37° C, both before implantation, and (3) at room temperature after explantation. The relation is linear and the temperature influence is small

resistance, the resistance of the strain gauge elements versus plate was checked before each reading using a Megohm-meter. If the resistance values fell below one Megohm, further measurements were considered to be unreliable. Most often such defects in insulation resulted from distal wire breakage, which made it possible to obtain a final reading at termination of the experiment following shortening of the wires.

The bridge amplifier used was a type Tepic Indicator IT 1. Zero-constancy and sensibility of the amplifier were tested before each measurement using a standard precision calibrator (Calibrator for strain indications Peekel type C 111).

After the *in vitro* calibrations were done an initial measurement was made during surgery at implantation. The protocol consisted of the following steps:

- Determination of the zero-point before fixation of the plate.
- Measurement of the zero-point, respecting the bending effect, after each one of the inner two screws was driven home.
- Continuous registration of the resulting axial compression force during insertion of all additional screws.
- Measurement of the total force in relation to the zero-point with bending-effect after all screws in both plates were driven home.

The first postoperative reading of the *static* longitudinal compression was made 15 minutes after termination of the surgical intervention. This measurement was repeated on the recumbent animal in right lateral position daily during the first postoperative week, twice during the second postoperative week and at weekly intervals thereafter. *Dynamic* compression forces were measured on the walking animal prior to explantation (see p. 13).

At explantation all steps of the intraoperative protocol were repeated in reverse order.

2.3.3. Measurement of Torque of the Screws

Driving home a screw causes a transverse compression within the bone. A comparison of the values at onset and end of the experiment gives information regarding a possible loosening of the implants.

Since transverse compression and torque exerted when screws are driven home are related linearly [5], we restricted ourselves simply to the measurement of torque in these experiments. This was done using a special screw driver equipped with strain gauge elements.

At explantation, two types of torque measurements were conducted: The initial torque when the screw fastening was first released ("torque of loosening") and subsequently the "torque of extraction". The "torque of loosening" is caused by the friction resistance between plate and screw as well as between screw thread and bone, when the screw is first loosened. The "torque of extraction" is registered after the screw has made the first one-half turn and represents the resistance between screw thread and bone only. By considering the two components one has an idea of the force with which the plate is pressed against the bone.

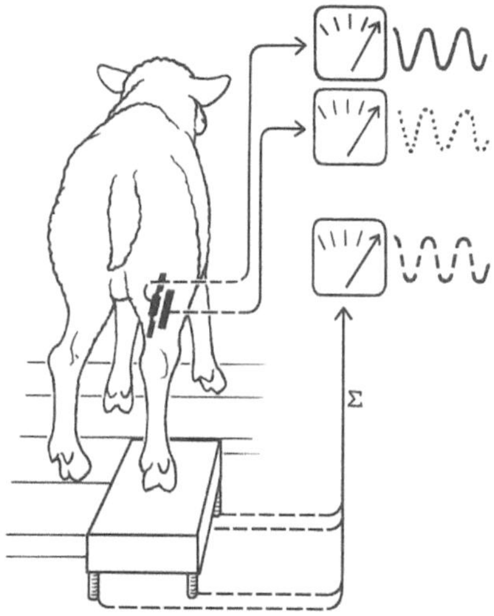

Fig. 11. Measurement of the forces while walking (loading test): The forces exerted between hoof and ground when loading the leg are measured using an electronic platform with piezo elements. Simultaneous registration of the forces through the implanted gauge plates offered a very sensitive test for early recognition of loosening of an implant. Comparative measurements of the forces exerted between hoof and ground through both hind legs very reliably showed even minimal degrees of diminished weight bearing!

2.3.4. Measurement of Weight Bearing (Force between Hoof and Ground)

The force exerted by the walking animal between the loaded extremity and the ground can be measured electronically. This force can be related to the stress transmitted by the implanted gauge plates.

The animals were conducted over a platform[6] which was on a level with a footpath and was rigidly connected with four piezo-electric elements. The force plate itself demonstrated no deformation when loaded due to its own inherent elastic properties. Therefore the total vertical force placed on the foot plate was registered by the piezo-electric elements, and the electrical signal from these elements was then transmitted to a charge-amplifier (Kistler 568) and passed to a multichannel-ink recorder (Watanabe Multicorder type MC 611). Simultaneous registration of the loading force between hoof and ground and of the impulses transmitted by the implanted gauge plates (group "compression with two gauge plates") showed the time correlation of the two forces (Fig. 11). In addition to the curves obtained while the animal was walking over the platform, recordings were taken of the standing animal when the extremity was loaded by induced weight displacement, accomplished when the physician monitor caused the animal to unweight one leg completely displacing the weight onto the leg being investigated. In some cases the curves obtained with this second method showed the interplay of forces more clearly and were then selected for illustration (Figs. 29–32).

The measurements of the forces at walking were made in all animals at the end of the experimental period of 8 weeks. In group "compression with one plate" and "no compression with one plate" additional measurements of the peak force when loading the extremity were made on the electronic scale at weekly intervals (loading test). Comparing the results of both hind legs, one had a sensitive test for recognition of even minimal unweighting of the operated extremity.

[6] Developed in collaboration with the firm Kistler, Winterthur-CH.

2.3.5. Infection and Control of Infectious Process

Six to eight days after surgery, when wound repair was well advanced, a known number of staphylococci were injected locally into the area of oste-

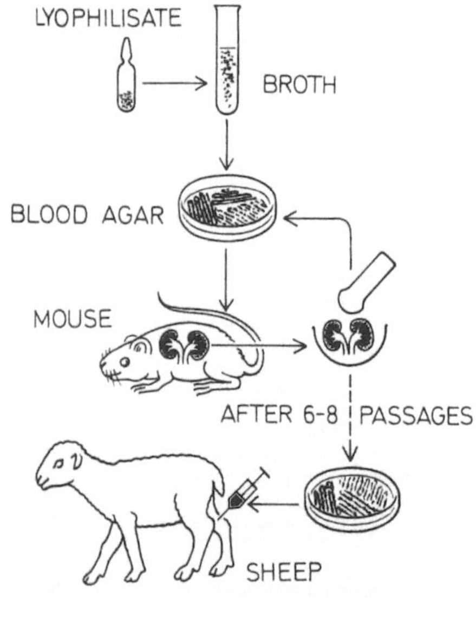

Fig. 12. Conditioning of the staphylococci for infection of the sheep in group "compression with two gauge plates": Staphylococci isolated from a human focus have been lyophilised. After suspension of this lyophilisate the virulence of the germs was maintained by blood agar and mice passages. After 5–8 such passages the sheep were infected with a bacterial suspension prepared on blood agar plates. Bacteria counts were performed in aliquot samples conserved at −28° C (see page 15)

otomy. The bacterial strain used had been isolated from a human staphylococcal infection. After several passages over blood agar plates and mice the bacteria were injected into the animals of group "compression with two gauge plates". The sheep developed local fistulae, from which organisms were isolated which were used to infect the animals of the groups "compression with one plate" and "no compression with one plate". Swabs from all fistulae were examined repeatedly for their bacterial content. Where no local secretions were available deep punctures were performed from the area of osteotomy. If the examinations were negative for bacteria, the injection of germs was repeated.

The strain of *staphylococcus aureus* used produced penicillinase and reacted with the bacteriophages 47/53/54/75 of the international phage set for typing. 2.2×10^8 lyophilised germs of this strain were suspended in 1 ml of thioglycollate broth (BBL) and incubated at 37° C over a 24 hour period. This culture was used to innoculate blood agar plates (Fig. 12). After incubation over 24–48 hours (37° C), the colonies grown were suspended in 1 ml of 0.9% NaCl solution. Dosages of 0.1 and 0.2 ml of this suspension were injected into one of the tail veins of SPF (specific pathogen free) mice of the strain NMRI. 24–48 hours later, mice which were evidently sick were killed and their kidneys excised and homogenised in 3 ml 0.9% NaCl solution. 1–5 drops of this suspension were put on blood agar plates and incubated at 37° C. 24–48 hours later the layer of bacteria grown was suspended in physiological NaCl solution and again injected into one of the tail veins of mice. The combined agar-/mice passages served for conservation of the germ virulence. During the agar-mice passages the characteristics of the bacterial cultures were tested continuously by gram-stains of the kidney homogenates as well as agar suspensions. Only those agar plates which showed the pigmentation, haemolysis and morphology of colonies typical for our strain were used for further cultivation.

After five to eight such passages the germs of the agar plates were suspended in 1 ml of a 0.9% NaCl solution, the suspension of several plates pooled and these then injected into the sheep of group "compression with two gauge plates". One portion of the bacterial pool was frozen at −28° C until bacterial counts could be performed. The local injection of the germ suspensions, done on the sixth to eighth postoperative day, was accomplished as follows:

— The sheep was placed in a right lateral recumbent position. In this position the implants of the osteotomised right tibia could be easily palpated through the skin.
— The skin over that area was disinfected several times with Desogen.
— 1 ml of the suspension was injected directly onto the bone near the osteotomy via an oblique puncture leading from a proximal external point to a distal internal location between the two gauge chambers of the two separate plates.
— The point of entry was then covered with Nobecutan spray and held under manual

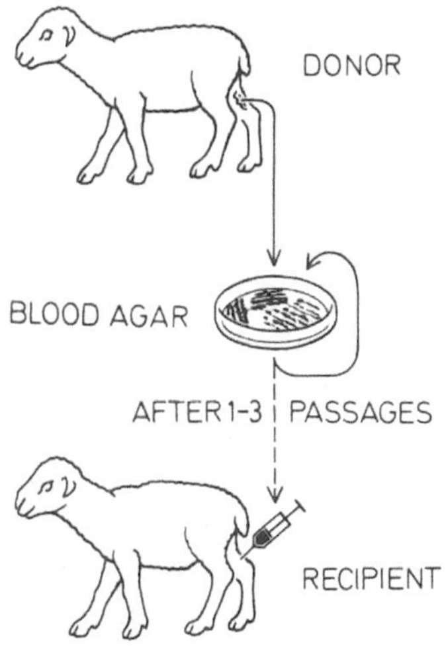

Fig. 13. Preparation of the staphylococcal suspension used to infect the sheep of groups "compression with one plate" and "no compression with one plate": The staphylococci used for the infection of these sheep were isolated from local fistula of the infected animals in group "compression with two gauge plates". The pus was cultured on blood agar plates. After 1–3 such passages the inoculum was prepared and aliquot samples conserved until counting of the bacteria was performed

compression using a sponge for a period of 5–10 minutes.

— The animals were thereafter allowed to move freely.

The animals in group "compression with one plate" and "no compression with one plate" were infected using the germs isolated from the pus of a sheep in group "compression with two gauge plates" (Fig. 13). The pus contained a pure staphylococcal culture as shown by gram-stain as well as the cultural characteristics. The phage type corresponded to the initial strain type 47/53/54/75. 24–72 hours prior to the infection of these sheep, the pus was isolated from the fistula and incubated on blood agar plates at 37° C. The colonies grown within 24 hours were suspended in 1 ml of 0.9% NaCl solution for each plate. Some of the animals were infected using this particular suspension, while in some cases the bacteria suspended went through two additional 24 hour passages on blood agar plates. This difference was caused by the fact that not all sheep were operated on simultaneously. Aliquot samples of the suspensions used for infection were kept at −28° C until germ counts were performed. The technique of infection was the same as described above (see p. 14).

Bacteriologic examination of the local secretions was made in all three groups, once between the second and fourth postoperative week and once in the sixth week. Where no fistula was present, a deep puncture was performed in the osteotomy zone. Of the material obtained gram-stains were made and broth tubes, as well as blood agar and McConkey plates inoculated for incubation. If staphylococcus grew within 24–48 hours, the plates were sent to the University Institute for Medical Microbiology in Zürich-CH, for phage typing. If other bacteria grew, which could not be easily identified in our laboratory, a second evaluation was made in the University Institute for Veterinary Bacteriology in Zürich-CH. If no clinical signs of infection were present early in the fourth week, and/or if the bacterial examination at that time showed only minimal or no staphylococcal growth, a second injection of staphylococci was performed. These organisms came from the same donor animal, but were kept in physiological saline solution at −28° C for conservation over 16–21 days. With this particular suspension, we were unable to institute an infection in our shep. Therefore 6–11 days later, a third injection of bacteria was given. This time, fresh bacteria recovered from the abscesses of another still available donor in group "compression with two gauge plates", were used for injection. These staphylococci were found to be identical with the original strain when examined by phage typing. Preparation of the inoculum as well as the technique of injection was done as described before.

The bacterial counts of the different suspensions used for infection were done by phase-contrast microscopy in a Thoma-counting chamber after fine dispersion by ultrasound.

2.3.6. Radiologic Examination

2.3.6.1. Plain Film X-Rays

The follow-up studies were done on the recumbent animal using the antero-posterior and medio-lateral direction of the X-ray beam. After an immediate postoperative control following surgery, the examination was repeated at 2 week intervals. (Technical details: 52–56 KV, 12 mAs, 70 cm focal distance, aluminium-filter of 3.0 mm diameter, Curix Special[7] film in a cassette with intensifying foil—Siemens Special). After explantation of the bone, high resolution X-ray films were taken using a Faxitron 804[8] apparatus. (Technical data: 56 KVP, 900 mAs, fine-focus tube, aluminium filter of 1.0 mm diameter, Structurix D4 film, no intensifying foil).

The X-ray films were reviewed independently by three radiologists and three bone surgeons. Special attention was directed to those criteria on which they based their diagnosis of osteitis in clinical situations, that is: *osteolysis, sequestrum, callus formation, sclerosis* and *fracture line* width as well as sharpness.

2.3.6.2. Microangiography

Using contrast media, the vascular tree can best be visualised on appropriate microscopic sections. Application of Indian Ink facilitates recognition of very small intraosseous vessels on light microscopy.

At termination of the experiments in the ninth week, 500 ml of Dextran 40 (Rheomacrodex) were infused via the external jugular vein. The femoral artery and vein were dissected free under anaesthesia. A polyethylene catheter was passed into the artery and then the vein was incised. After injection of 5000 IU of Heparin in 9 ml of Ringer solution and 150 mg of Ronicol (3 ml) through the arterial cannula, the extremity was perfused with 100 ml of Indian Ink (warmed to 37° C) using a constant infusion pump set at 120 mm Hg. Care was taken to avoid entry of air into the system. The perfusion was continued using 200 ml of a 20% barium sulphate solution (Micropaque), filtered through a net with 20 μm pore size (modified after the method of RHINELANDER *et al.* [93]). Therafter the tibia was explanted and kept at −28° C.

Subsequent to this and after explantation of the bone, additional steps were accomplished in the course of the histological preparation (see p. 18). In this manner, a longitudinal cut of 1 mm in diameter was taken from the decalcified medial bone segment which was embedded in methyl methacrylate. The microangiographic pictures were obtained in the Faxitron 804 apparatus at a 30 min. exposure time, 19–22 KVP tube power and 3 mA current intensity. Kodak High Resolution Plates Sp 0650 and Spectroscopic Plates 649-0 were used as films.

2.3.6.3. Microradiography

The microradiographic examination gives the best three-dimensional view of new bone apposition and old bony structures. The differentiation between new and old bone is based on the difference in X-ray absorption due to the difference in calcium content.

At the time of bone preparation for histology, 100 μm thick cuts were made from the osteotomy region (see p. 17). These non-decalcified saw cuts were exposed to X-rays in the Faxitron 804 apparatus. (Technical data: 19–22 KVP tube power, 3 mA current intensity, 30 min. exposure time, Kodak High Resolution Plates Sp 0650 film photographed at 10 fold magnification).

2.3.7. Polychrome Sequential Labelling and Histological Preparation

Time sequence and the 3-dimensional aspects of bone reconstruction can best be studied by use of fluorochromes, injected at given intervals and subsequently deposited in new bone. From the explanted bone fine saw cuts were made for micro-

[7] Produced by Agfa Gevaert.
[8] Produced by Field Emission Corp., Oregon, USA.

Table 2. Polychrome sequential labelling of new bone formation using fluorochromes

Symbol	Time	Substance	Dosage (mg/kg BW)
CB_1	2nd week	calcein blue	30
CB_2	3rd week	calcein blue	30
XO	4th week	xylenol orange	90
C_1	5th week	calcein green	20
C_2	6th week	calcein green	20
AC	7th week	alizarin complexone	30

scopic study of new bone formation, as well as fine sections of decalcified segments showing cell formation.

The labels were injected in 2% Na-bicarbonate solution subcutaneously after sterile filtration. Table 2 lists sequence, material and dosage of the fluorochromes injected [87, 88, 90].

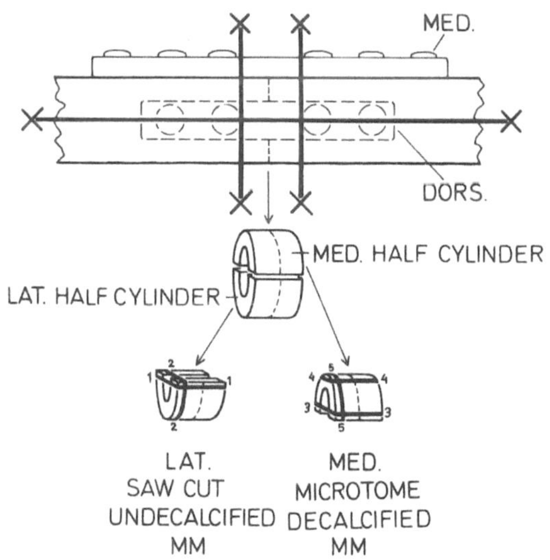

Fig. 14. Sectional planes used for histological evaluation of the explanted bone: The midsegment in between the inner two screws was cut out and severed into a lateral and medial half-cylinder. The mode of preparation used is marked under each bone segment (*e.g.* MM = methyl methacrylate). The numbers listed characterise the sectional planes described in the text

The histological work up did not immediately follow explantation. Therefore, the explanted bones were rapidly frozen down to −50° C and kept at −28° C thereafter. The midsegment of the bone between the inner two screws, containing the osteotomy site, was excised utilising a circular saw with cooled blade (liquid nitrogen). Figure 14 illustrates the location of this and the following cuts. The numbers listed will be used in the text to characterise a specific sectional plane. First the midsegment was cut into a medial half-cylinder, formerly covered by the 6-hole plate, and a lateral half-cylinder. These two parts were prepared as follows:

Lateral half-cylinder:

— Dehydration using increasing alcohol concentrations (40%, 80%, 96%, 100% for a duration of one day each); thereafter treatment with xylol (1–2 days).
— Embedding in methyl methacrylate (MM); the section is placed into stabilised monomer MM for the duration of 1 day. A mixture of 100 ml MM and 2 g benzoyl peroxide (dehydrated over calcium chloride) is then added and maintained with constant agitation for better permeation of the solution. The section is finally placed into a mixture of 100 ml MM and 4 g benzoyl peroxide and

2.5 ml Plastoid and kept in a water bath at 34° C for polymerisation (modified method of SCHENK [100]).

- Longitudinal (1) and transverse (2) cuts.
- Further thinning by means of grinding of these cuts in between two glass plates with roughened surfaces to a thickness of 80 μm.

These non-stained saw cuts served for light and fluorescent microscopy study as well as microradiographic studies.

Medial half-cylinder:

- Fixing in 40% ethanol for several days.
- Decalcification using 15% formic acid over 2 days.
- Dehydration using increasing concentrations of alcohol, then xylol.
- Embedding in methyl methacrylate.
- Longitudinal (3 and 4) as well as transverse cuts (5) of 6 μm thickness using a Zeiss-hard-cut microtome.
- Staining with haemalaune-eosin (Goldner-Masson Trichrome) and using the Gallamine-Giemsa method (described by BURKHARDT [13].

These decalcified microtome cuts were used to study the fine structural elements of the bone and soft tissue cells. 1 mm thick cuts from the remaining portion of the medial half-cylinder served for microangiographic studies.

2.4. Summary of the Experimental Protocol (Fig. 15)

Transverse osteotomies of the sheep tibia have been stabilised using different implants. After one week, staphylococci have been injected into the osteotomy zone. Local bacterial examinations were made twice between the second and sixth postoperative week. In a few cases with negative or only slightly positive bacterial cultures of staphylococci, repetition of the injection of bacteria was required. Loading of the extremity operated was tested clinically and by electronic balance. In one group these measurements of the loading forces were combined with the registration of the force transmission through the implants before sacrificing the animals. Interfragmentary compression was measured in one group first during surgery and then periodically as well as at explantation. At termination of the experiments (9th week), bacteriologic control examinations were made in all animals before filling the vessels of the extremity with contrast media. The measurements of torque first made at implantation were repeated when the screws were removed. Histological examinations followed.

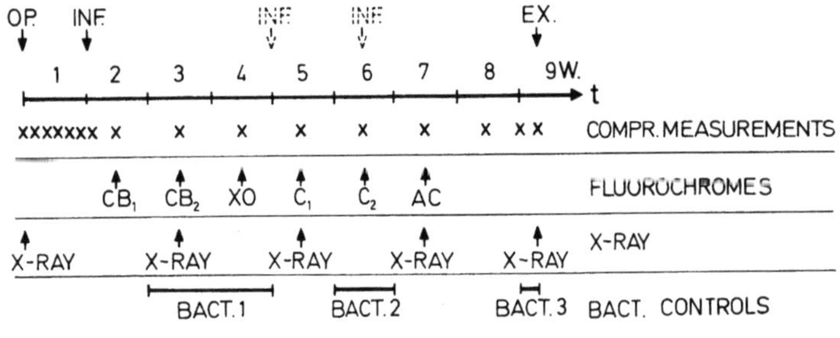

Fig. 15. Synopsis of the experimental protocol: On the x-axis the time intervals (t) are given in weeks (W). OP: Operation with osteotomy and internal fixation, measurement of the torque of the screws. INF: Local injections of bacteria and eventual reinfections. EX: Explantation with measurement of the loading force between hoof and ground, angiography, registration of torque and interfragmentary compression. X: Measurement of interfragmentary compression in group "compression with two gauge plates". CB_{1-2}, XO; C_{1-2}, AC: Application of fluorochromes (see Table 2). X-RAY: X-ray controls. BACT. 1–3: Bacteriologic controls

Results

3.1. General Aspects

All animals recovered from the surgical procedure without complications. One sheep died in the third postoperative week from asphyxia when its neck became trapped between the bars of the box. Three animals died from systemic diseases, whereby in 2 cases a systemic spread from the local infectious process could not be excluded with certainty. Two animals of the group "no compression with one plate" sustained a fracture of the operated extremity within the first postoperative week. Table 3 lists all ani-

Table 3. Synopsis of all animals excluded from the experiment during the time-course of the study: Six sheep had to be excluded from the study. Three animals died before the local injections of staphylococci were made, two before the bacterial controls of the wound were done.
1) Death before injection of staphylococci. 2) Bacteriologic examination not made or not of conclusive value

DAYS postop.	SHEEP No.	GROUP	PATHOL. ANAT. FINDINGS	BACTERIOLOGY WOUND	BACTERIOLOGY ORGANS
6	1453	"Compression with one plate"	Heart: focal degeneration Sarcosporids +++ Spleen: hyperemia Liver: enlarged	1)	Liver: E.coli Spleen: E.coli Musculat.: E.coli Cl.Welchii
6	1954	"No compression with one plate"	Tibia fracture	1)	2)
7	1459	"No compression with one plate"	Tibia fracture	1)	2)
16	18	"Compression with two gauge plates"	Lungs: hyperemia +++, edema + Heart: Sarcosporids +++ degeneration + Lymphn.: edema ++, plasma cells ++ Spleen: hyperemia +++	Staph. aur. haemolyt., Gram ⊖ rods, Streptococci type A	Liver: E.coli
19	2298	"No compression with one plate"	Lungs: hyperemia +++, edema +++ Heart: hyperemia, edema, haemorrhages Liver: hyperemia N.B. caught between bars of stable → asphyxia	2)	2)
21	22	"Compression with one plate"	Lungs: edema +++, hyperemia +++ Liver: leeches, focal infiltrates, chron. cholangitis Lymphn.: induration Kidney: acute nephrosis	2)	Liver: E.coli Spleen: E.coli Kidney: E.coli

mals mentioned which had to be excluded from the study throughout the experimental period due to general or local complications. 19 animals, therefore, participated further and completed the study—8 sheep in group "compression with two gauge plates", 5 sheep in group "compression with one plate" and 6 sheep in group "no compression with one plate". In one of these animals the experiment was terminated early (in the seventh postoperative week) due to severe deterioration of the general condition. An acute, purulent, necrotising encephalitis manifest by scattered foci of involvement was found in this sheep at autopsy; thus a listeriosis could not be excluded. Other diseases transiently observed in the animals included: non-specific cough in one, purulent conjunctivitis on three occasions, hyper-tachypnea in one case, difficulty with equilibrium once and "claw-rot" once. All these healed within a few days, even though these animals also received no antibiotics.

The animals started walking at the earliest 30 min. after surgery, but never later than 12 hours postoperatively. Some sheep limped during a variable period of time. Wound healing was uncomplicated until the end of the first week. Following the local injections of staphylococci, 16 out of the 19 animals developed secondary disturbances of wound healing with fistulae. The bacterial examinations of the local secretions were positive for staphylococci or, in several instances, other organisms of a mixed infection type in all sheep, including 4 animals which were revaccinated.

Histological evaluation showed that 18 out of 19 animals had reached bony union of the osteotomy within 8 weeks.

In the following more detailed description of the results, the observations made on each sheep will be listed individually. This allows the reader to follow individual cases for specific information.

3.2. Local Infection

The bacterial content of the suspensions used to infect the sheep is listed in Table 4. In the batches used for the first four sheep (739, 1297, 878, 741), the determination was not possible for technical reasons. The numbers of bacteria used varied only minimally between values of $3.1–12.9 \times 10^{10}$.

The characteristics of the infectious disease are summarised for each group in Tables 5–7.

Table 4. List of bacterial counts of the suspensions used to infect the sheep: Most suspensions served to infect several animals. The counts of the different solutions varied only slightly

SUSPENSION	RECIPIENT ANIMAL	BACTERIAL COUNT 10^{10}/ml
I	15 / 821 / 16	4.5
II	785 / 847	3.5
III	21 / 1829	4.9
IV	2287	12.9
V	23/24/2265/4214/4213	3.1
VI	279 / 1008	5.7

Table 5. The results of bacteriologic examination and clinical as well as autopsy findings in group "compression with two gauge plates"

SHEEP No.	1st. BACTERIOLOGIC CONTROL 2-4 week	2nd. BACTERIOLOGIC CONTROL 5-6 week	3rd. BACTERIOLOGIC CONTROL exitus (9th. week)	PHAGE TYPE a) at 1st. bact. control b) at 3rd. bact. control	Clinical or autopsy findings
739	Staph. aureus	Staph. aureus	Staph. aureus	a) 6/47/53/54/75/83A b) 6/42E/47/53/54/75	calor, limping, large callus mass
1297	Staph. aureus	Staph. aureus	Staph. aureus (few), Staph. epidermidis	a) 6/42E/47/53/54/75/83A b) not typeable	fistula 3-9 weeks
878	Staph. aureus (few), ß-hemolyt. Streptococci	Staph. aureus (few), ß-hemolyt. Streptococci	Staph. aureus (few), ß-hemolyt. Streptococci, Neisseria	a) 3A/3C b) 3A	abscess 4-9 weeks
741	Staph. aureus	Staph. aureus (few), ß-hemolyt. Streptococci	Staph. aureus	a) 6/47/53/54/75/83A b) 6/42E/47/53/54/75	fistula 3-9 weeks
15	Staph. aureus, Pneumococci, Gram. neg. rods	Staph. aureus, ß-hemolyt. Streptococci	Staph. aureus, ß-hemolyt. Streptococci	a) 6/47/54 b) 6/42E/47/53/54/75	fistula 2-9 weeks
821	Staph. aureus	Staph. aureus	Staph. aureus	a) 6/47/53/54/75/83A b) 6/42E/47/53/54/75	fistula 6-9 weeks no signs of infection before
16	Staph. aureus	Staph. aureus	Staph. aureus	a) 6/47/53/54/75/83A b) 6/42E/47/53/54/75/83A	fistula in 3rd. week, thereafter only calor, 2 deep abscesses at sacrifice
2287	Staph. aureus	Staph. aureus	no growth	a) 6/47/53/54/75/83A b) ---	fistula after 7th. week, calor before, limping

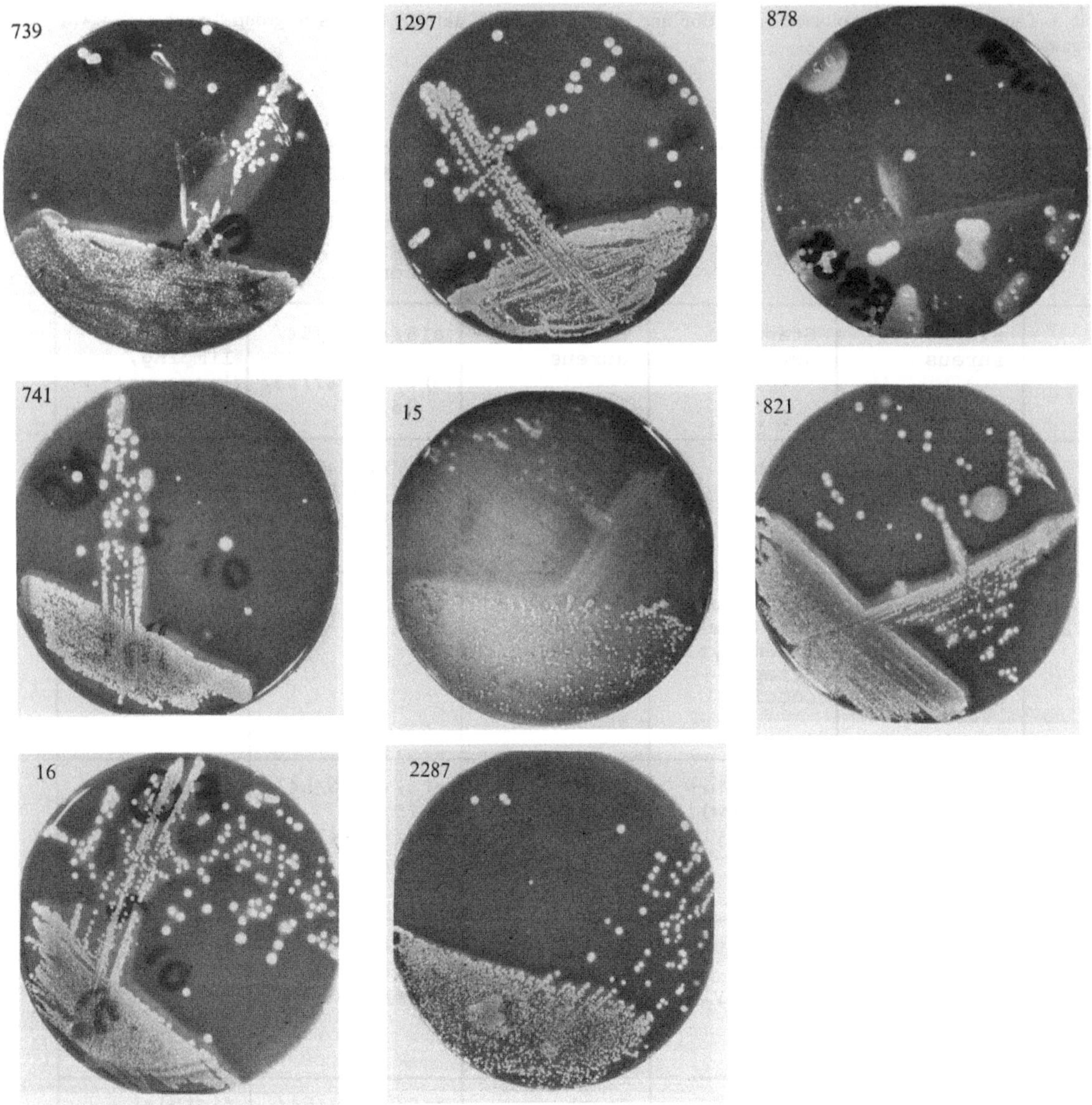

Fig. 16. Synopsis of a bacteriologic control in group "compression with two gauge plates": The blood agar plates of one of the bacteriologic examinations showing that all animals had haemolytic staphylococci in their osteotomy region

Group *"compression with two gauge plates"* (Table 5, Fig. 16):

Bacteria. Three sheep (739, 821, 16) showed pure staphylococcal monoinfections until sacrifice. In four animals (1297, 878, 741, 15) *staphylococcus epidermidis*, *β*-haemolytic streptococci, pneumococci, gram-negative rods and *neisseriae sp.* were additionally found. In one sheep (2287), the final culture was negative after two preceding cultures showing pure growth of *staphylococcus aureus.* Inasmuch as the phage type could be determined, it did not change when compared to the initial type [10] with the exception of the organisms found in one case (sheep 878), in which most likely a superinfection with another strain of staphylococci had occured.

Revaccination. Since all animals had positive cultures for staphylococci no additional injection of organisms was necessary.

Local Examination. The clinical signs of infection were clearly minor in those sheep with pure staphylococcal monoinfection, and in the case with the negative final bacteriological examination when compared to the cases exhibiting mixed bacterial growth. In the latter cases deep abscesses and heavily secreting fistulae occurred. (*e.g.* Fig. 17).

Systemic Spread of the Infectious Disease. One case of coughing (sheep 878) and one of conjunctivitis (sheep 741) could be looked upon as a complication of the local infectious process.

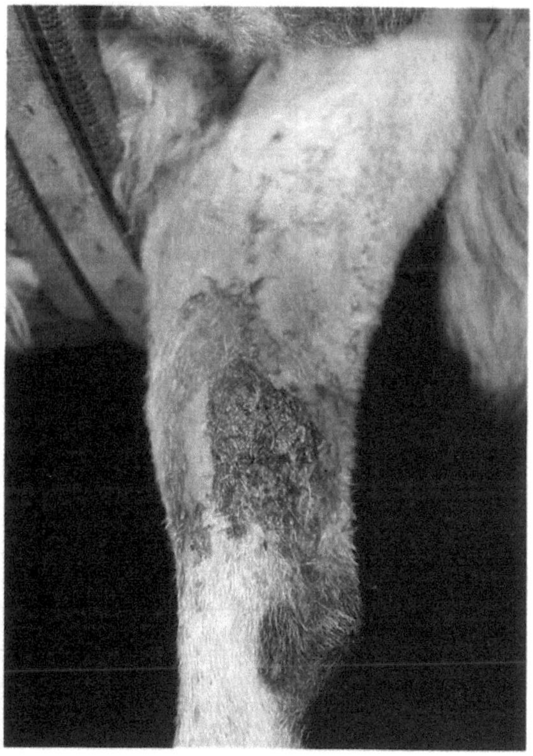

Fig. 17. Local aspect of one sheep of group "compression with two gauge plates": From the fourth week on, sheep 15 suffered from a profusely discharging fistula (mixed infection)

Group *"compression with one plate"* (Table 6, Fig. 18):

Bacteria. All sheep in this group showed mixed infections; in one sheep (2665) no staphylococci were found at explantation. The germs most commonly encountered associated with staphylococci were *E. coli* and *β*-haemolytic streptococci; more seldom *staphylococcus epidermidis* and *corynebacterium pyogenes* were seen. No change in the staphylococcal phage type was noted.

Revaccination. Two out of the five animals (sheep 23 and 2665) showed only minimal or no staphylococcal growth at first examination. After a first revaccination using deep frozen bacteria (see p. 15) the bacteriologic control examination was again negative. After a second revaccination, both animals developed massive mixed bacterial growth, in one of which staphylococci were absent.

Local Examination. All animals of this group exhibited fistulae, which remained open in four animals (279, 23, 2665, 4213) from the third or fourth week on, while the fistula of sheep 1829 soon disappeared spontaneously.

Systemic Spread of the Infectious Disease. The early death of one sheep (23) in the seventh week seems most likely to be a consequence of the

Table 6. The results of bacteriologic examination and clinical as well as autopsy local findings in group "compression with one plate": Sheep 23 died in the 7th week, so that a final bacteriologic study was made in the 6th week instead of the routine second examination. 1) Examination not performed

SHEEP No.	1st. BACTERIOLOGIC CONTROL 4th. week	2nd. BACTERIOLOGIC CONTROL 6th. week	3rd. BACTERIOLOGIC CONTROL exitus (9th. week)	PHAGE TYPE a) at 1st. bact. control b) at 3rd. bact. control	Clinical or autopsy findings
1829	Staph. aureus, Staph. epidermidis (few)	Staph. aureus	Staph. aureus, Staph. epidermidis (few)	a) 80/6/42E/47/53/54/75/83A b) 6/42E/47/53/54/75	fistula in 5th. week, rubor, calor, chron. granulation tissue
279	Staph. aureus, ß-hemol. Streptococci (few)	Staph. aureus, ß-hemol. Streptococci	Staph. aureus, C. pyogenes, E. coli	a) 6/42E/47/53/54/75/83A b) 6/42E/47/53/54/75/83A	fistula 4-9 weeks
23	ß-hemol. Streptococci, E. coli	1)	Staph. aureus, E. coli, C. pyogenes	a) --- b) 3A/6/42E/47/53/54/75	fistula 3-9 weeks
2665	Staph. aureus (few), C. pyogenes, ß-hemol. Streptococci	C. pyogenes, ß-hemol. Streptococci	C. pyogenes, E. coli	a) 6/42E/47/53/54/75 b) ---	fistula 3-9 weeks
4213	Staph. aureus	Staph. aureus, Coliform organisms	Staph. aureus, E. coli	a) 6/42E/47/53/54/83A b) 6/42E/47/53/54/75	fistula 3-9 weeks

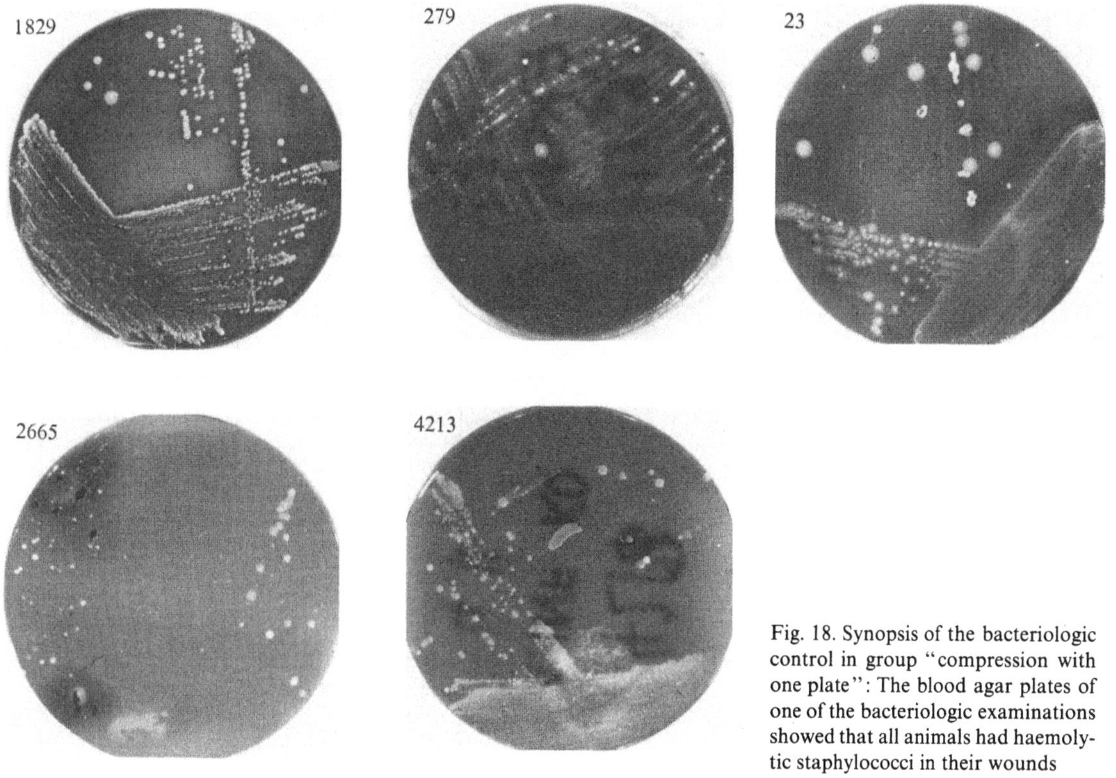

Fig. 18. Synopsis of the bacteriologic control in group "compression with one plate": The blood agar plates of one of the bacteriologic examinations showed that all animals had haemolytic staphylococci in their wounds

infection. The wound of this animal was colonised with *E. coli* from the fourth week on and after repeated injections of staphylococci, also with *staphylococcus aureus*. At autopsy the sheep presented a purulent, necrotising encephalitis; acute, purulent glomerulonephritis; myocarditis; and focal purulent infiltrations of the lymph nodes. All of these findings could have resulted from an *E. coli* sepsis, even though *E. coli* could not be cultured from the bloodstream. The veterinary pathologists expressed a suspicion of listeriosis.

Group *"no compression with one plate"* (Table 7, Fig. 19):

Bacteria: One sheep (785) exhibited a pure staphylococcal monoinfection throughout the period of observation. In all other animals *E. coli,* diphtheroids, *C. pyogenes,* fungi and *staphylococcus epidermidis* were found in addition. The phage type of the staphylococci was unchanged.

Revaccination. At first examination one animal (1008) had no bacterial growth and one other sheep (21) had no staphylococci. After two *re*injections, staphylococci were found abundantly in these, as in all other animals.

Local Examination. Four sheep (24, 4214, 785, 847) presented abscesses with fistulae after the third or fourth week. Both animals with repeated

Table 7. The results of bacteriologic examination and clinical as well as autopsy findings in group "no compression with one plate"

SHEEP No.	1st BACTERIOLOGIC CONTROL 4th. week	2nd. BACTERIOLOGIC CONTROL 6th. week	3rd. BACTERIOLOGIC CONTROL exitus (9th. week)	PHAGE TYPE a) at 1st. bact. control b) at 3rd. bact. control	Clinical or autopsy findings
21	no growth	mixed germs	Staph. aureus	a) --- b) not typeable	rubor, calor, granulation tissue
1008	Staph. aureus (few), mixed germs	Staph. aureus	Staph. aureus, E. coli	a) not typeable b) 6/42E/47/53/54/75	calor, rubor 5-6 weeks deep abscess
24	Staph. aureus	Staph. aureus, diphth. rods, fungi	Staph. aureus, C. pyogenes, E. coli	a) 6/42E/47/53/54/75 b) 6/42E/47/53/54/75	fistula 3-9 weeks
4214	Staph. aureus	Staph. aureus, Staph. epidermidis	Staph. aureus, E. coli	a) 6/42E/47/53/54/75 b) 6/42E/47/53/54/75	fistula 4-9 weeks
785	Staph. aureus	Staph. aureus	Staph. aureus	a) 6/42E/47/53/54/75 b) 6/42E/47/53/54/75/83A	fluctuation 4-8 weeks, fistula 8-9 weeks
847	Staph. aureus	Staph. aureus, diphth. rods	Staph. aureus (few), C. pyogenes, E. coli	a) 6/47/53/54/75 b) not typeable	fistula 3-9 weeks

bacterial injections had only minor local signs of infection in face of bacterial cultures which became positive. At explantation however, deep granulation tissue and pus were found over the implants.

Systemic Spread of the Infectious Disease. Two cases of conjunctivitis (sheep 21, 847), one of which was associated with hyper-tachypnea without additional symptoms, could be the result of spreading of the local infection. These symptoms cleared in a short time without treatment.

3.3. Interfragmentary Compression

The gauge plates which were implanted in group "compression with two gauge plates" for monitoring of interfragmentary pressure changes, had properties which will next be discussed.

Technical Remarks. In vitro calibration of the gauge plates showed a linear correlation between measured strain and axial force (see *e.g.* p. 12, Fig. 10). The temperature effects on the zero-level (Table 8) was minimal, amounting to

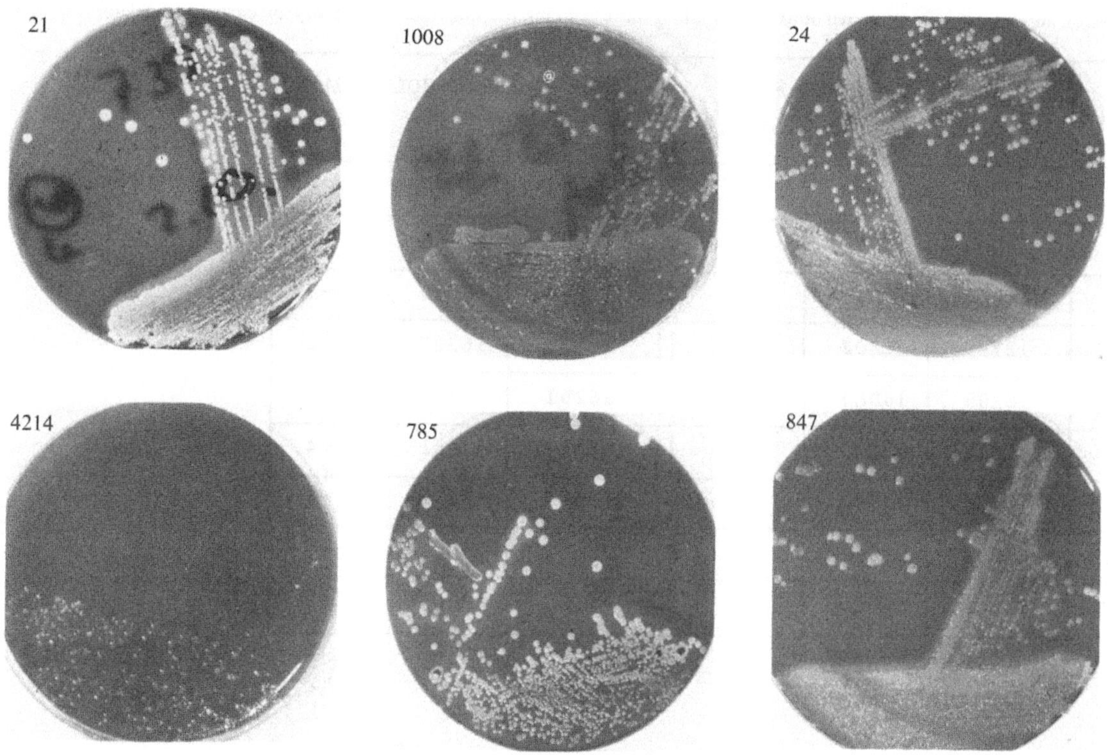

Fig. 19. Synopsis of a bacteriologic control in group "no compression with one plate": The blood agar plates of a bacteriologic control showing that haemolytic staphylococci were found in all animals, most commonly associated with other germs

$-2.35\ \mu/°C \pm 3.39$ SD, the effect on sensitivity (Table 9) being as little as $+0.17\ \mu/kp/°C \pm 0.10$ SD.

Before each measurement, the bridge amplifier was calibrated. The zero-point of the amplifier deviated less than 10 μ throughout the entire period of observation and the sensitivity showed no measurable change.

Bending of the plate at implantation to suit the bone surface caused no significant plastic deformation of the gauge chamber (Table 10). The elastic deformation of the plates as measured at implantation and explantation were considered when values for interfragmentary compression were measured. These values are listed in Table 11.

By the end of the surgical procedure the sum of axial compression measured in both plates varied in the eight animals between 98 and 220 kp. Individual values are available in Figs. 20–27. These values are clearly delineated in respect to zero-point sensitivity, elastic deformation and temperature influence, by relating them to the calibration which immediately preceded the tests. The compression forces still active at the termination of the experiments varied from 0 to 103 kp for the eight animals, and were again well defined by calibration immediately following explantation. The values obtained between implantation and explantation must be viewed as being dependent on alterations in zero-point and sensitivity occurring between the initial and terminal calibrations. These changes are listed in Tables 12 and 13. They are only minor changes when compared to the biologic variations due to muscle activity, etc.

Changes in Interfragmentary Compression (Figs. 20–27). In 15 out of 16 gauge plates reliable measurements could be made at the beginning and end of the experiment. In the one remaining plate, the wires required shortening so much fol-

Table 8. Influence of temperature on zero-point: The zero shifted only a little when measured at 22 ± 1° C and 37 ± 1° C. This difference in strain (μ) is converted into kp by taking into account the individual sensitivity of each gauge plate

SHEEP No.	ZERO-POINT 6-HOLE PLATE			ZERO-POINT 4-HOLE PLATE		
	22±1°C	37±1°C	DIFF.	22±1°C	37±1°C	DIFF.
	μ	μ	kp	μ	μ	kp
739	14031	13998	+5	16607	16626	-2
1297	14052	14007	+7	16409	16430	-3
878	12799	12802	-0	16379	16387	-1
741	16105	16087	+3	16251	16264	-1
15	15312	15298	+2	14087	14061	+4
821	14372	14352	+3	16348	16373	-3
16	14704	14761	-9	15682	15690	-1
2287	14608	14635	-4	15757	15764	-1

Table 9. Temperature effect on the sensitivity of the gauge plates: Sensitivity (μ/kp) represents the relationship between change in strain (μ) and axial force (kp). Only slight differences in sensitivity are found when measured at 22 ± 1° C and 37 ± 1° C. The percentage difference was calculated as deviation of the value at 22° C from the one at 37° C

SHEEP No.	6-HOLE PLATE			4-HOLE PLATE		
	22±1°C	37±1°C	DIFF.	22±1°C	37±1°C	DIFF.
	μ/kp	μ/kp	%	μ/kp	μ/kp	%
739	6.7	6.8	-2	9.5	9.7	-2
1297	6.8	6.8	0	7.2	7.4	-3
878	6.3	6.3	0	7.3	7.5	-3
741	6.9	7.0	-1	9.5	9.7	-2
15	6.8	7.0	-3	6.6	6.8	-3
821	6.6	6.8	-3	7.5	7.5	0
16	6.6	6.7	-1	8.3	8.8	-6
2287	6.8	6.9	-1	8.6	8.7	-1

Table 10. Plastic deformation due to bending of the plate to suit the bone surface: Bending of the implants caused no significant plastic deformation of the gauge chamber. The zero point measured *in vitro* at 37±1° C correlated well with the *in vivo* measurement at surgery. The difference is converted into kp to demonstrate the resulting effect more clearly

SHEEP	ZERO-POINT 6-HOLE PLATE			ZERO-POINT 4-HOLE PLATE		
	IN VITRO	INTRAOP.	DIFF.	IN VITRO	INTRAOP.	DIFF.
	μ	μ	kp	μ	μ	kp
739	13998	13995	0	16626	16630	0
1297	14007	13975	5	16430	16405	3
878	12802	12788	2	16387	16387	0
741	16087	16075	2	16264	16275	1
15	15298	15265	5	14061	14060	0
821	14352	14405	8	16373	16370	0
16	14761	14739	3	15690	15669	2
2287	14635	14617	3	15764	15760	0

Table 11. Elastic deformation of the plates at implantation and explantation: Driving home each one of the inner screws caused a temporary shift of the zero-point (elastic deformation). This difference is measured in μ and is caused by foreign forces; it can easily be converted into kp by taking into account the sensitivity of each plate. This bending influence is taken into account when compression measurements are made

SHEEP No.	ELASTIC BENDING FORCE 6-HOLE PLATE				ELASTIC BENDING FORCE 4-HOLE PLATE			
	IMPLANT.		EXPLANT.		IMPLANT.		EXPLANT.	
	μ	kp	μ	kp	μ	kp	μ	kp
739	-50	7	0	0	0	0	0	0
1297	-15	2	-33	5	0	0	0	0
878	-72	11	-45	7	0	0	+59	8
741	-58	8	-53	6	-63	7	-22	2
15	-25	4	-18	2	-20	3	-5	1
821	-80	12	-76	10	-8	1	-25	3
16	-100	15	-48	7	-5	1	-12	2
2287	-56	8	-30	4	-25	3	+15	2

Table 12. Zero shift during the experimental period: Determination of the zero-point at explantation shows good correlation with the values at implantation, when the changes in resistance due to the shortening of the electrical wires at explantation are considered. The difference is listed in kp taking into account the sensitivity of each plate

SHEEP	ZERO-POINT 6-HOLE PLATE			ZERO-POINT 4-HOLE PLATE		
	IMPLANT.	EXPLANT.	DIFF.	IMPLANT.	EXPLANT.	DIFF.
	μ	μ	kp	μ	μ	kp
739	13995	13936	-10	16630	16585	+5
1297	13975	13967	-1	16405	16359	+7
878	12788	12781	-1	16387	16357	+4
741	16075	16042	+5	16275	16245	+3
15	15265	15241	+4	14060	14041	-3
821	14405	14367	-6	16370	16317	+7
16	14739	14711	-5	15669	15650	+2
2287	14617	14587	-5	15760	15717	+5

Figs. 20–27. *In vivo* changes of interfragmentary compression in the sheep of group "compression with two gauge plates": ▷ The compression values of each individual plate as well as the sum of the two are presented. The values at the beginning and end of the experiment are well defined by the immediately preceeding or following calibrations. The values in between are subject to the minor variations in zero-point and sensitivity between implantation and explantation. Lines have been drawn through the individual points of determination. ▲Measurements of the 4-hole plate. ⌘Measurements of the 6-hole plate. ● Sum of the values of the two plates. --- A dotted line characterises sudden changes between two points of measurement; no exact localisation of the turning point is possible. Where the line is interrupted (broken wire) measurements were temporarily interrupted until the end of the experiment

Table 13. Changes in sensitivity between implantation and explantation: The load-strain diagrams obtained at implantation and explantation show good agreement of the sensitivity (μ/kp). The percentage difference was calculated as deviation of the value at explantation from the one at implantation

SHEEP	6-HOLE PLATE			4-HOLE PLATE		
	IMPLANT.	EXPLANT.	DIFF.	IMPLANT.	EXPLANT.	DIFF.
	μ/kp	μ/kp	%	μ/kp	μ/kp	%
739	6.7	6.2	-7	9.5	--*	--
1297	6.8	6.0	-12	7.2	6.6	-8
878	6.3	6.1	-3	7.3	7.6	+4
741	6.9	6.9	0	9.5	9.0	-5
15	6.8	6.1	-10	6.6	6.5	-2
821	6.6	6.4	-3	7.5	7.9	+4
16	6.6	5.7	-14	8.3	7.9	-5
2287	6.8	6.0	-12	8.6	8.1	-6

* The 4-hole plate of sheep 739 could not be recalibrated at the time of explantation due to a broken wire in the immediate neighbourhood of the gauge chamber.

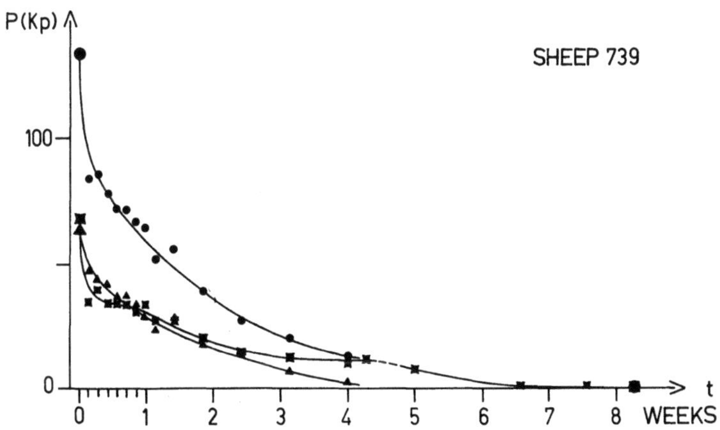

Fig. 20. *In vivo* changes of interfragmentary compression in sheep 739: After a steep initial decrease in both plates occurring during the first three days, compression in the 4-hole plate undergoes a continuous slow further reduction and reaches values around zero in the fourth week. Interfragmentary compression in the 6-hole plate shows a second rapid decrease in the fourth week and reaches zero in the sixth week

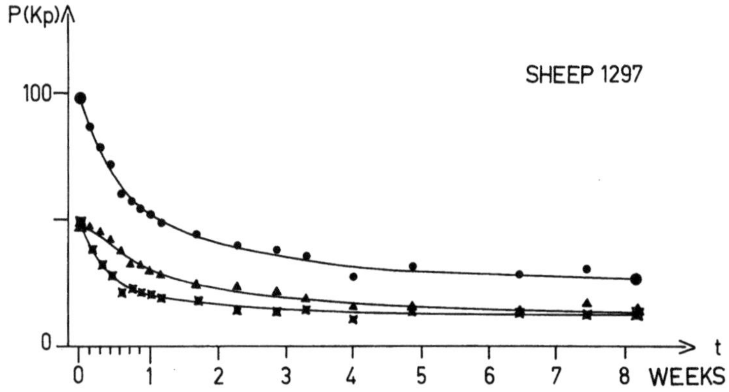

Fig. 21. *In vivo* changes of interfragmentary compression in sheep 1297: After an initial rapid drop in compression only a slight further decrease was observed

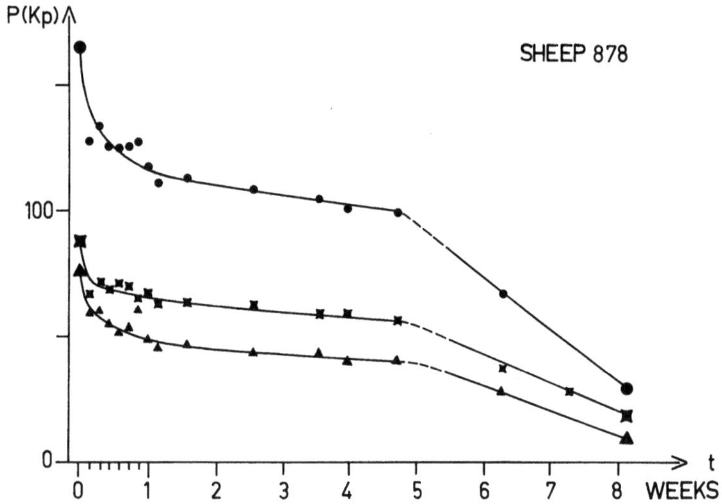

Fig. 22. *In vivo* changes in interfragmentary compression in sheep 878: There is a secondary steep decline in compression in the fourth week. The remaining total axial force at the end of eight weeks amounts to 29 kp

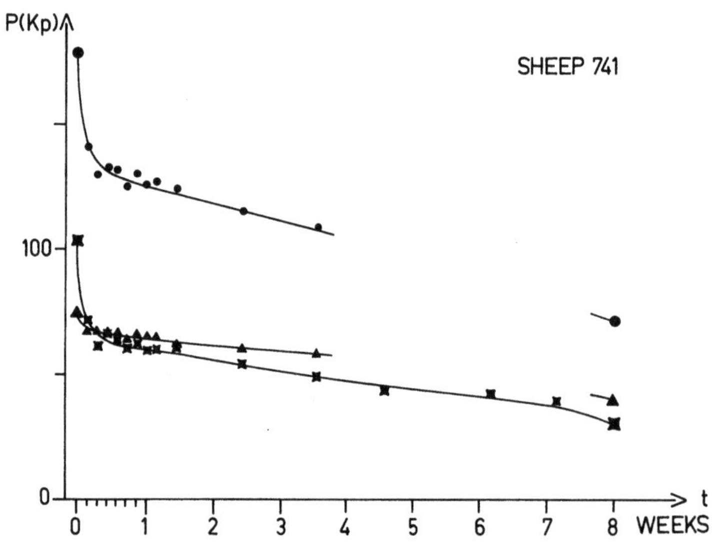

Fig. 23. *In vivo* changes in interfragmentary compression in sheep 741: After an initial pressure drop in both plates occurring within the first five days, a second phase of only slight further loss of compression is observed lasting until termination of the experiment. In the fourth week no further readings could be obtained from the 4-hole plate due to a broken wire. The final reading indicates that there was a slow further decrease in pressure during the given interval

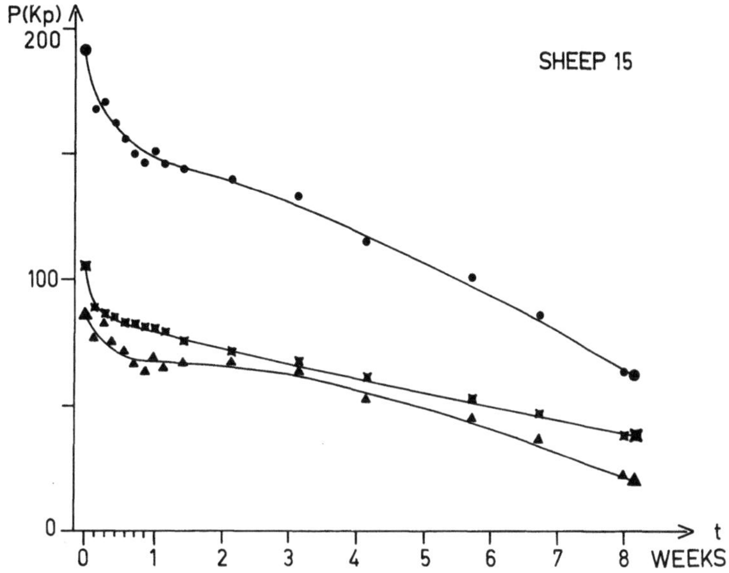

Fig. 24. *In vivo* changes of interfragmentary compression in sheep 15: Slow reduction in pressure with only a slight secondary drop in the 4-hole plate after the fourth week

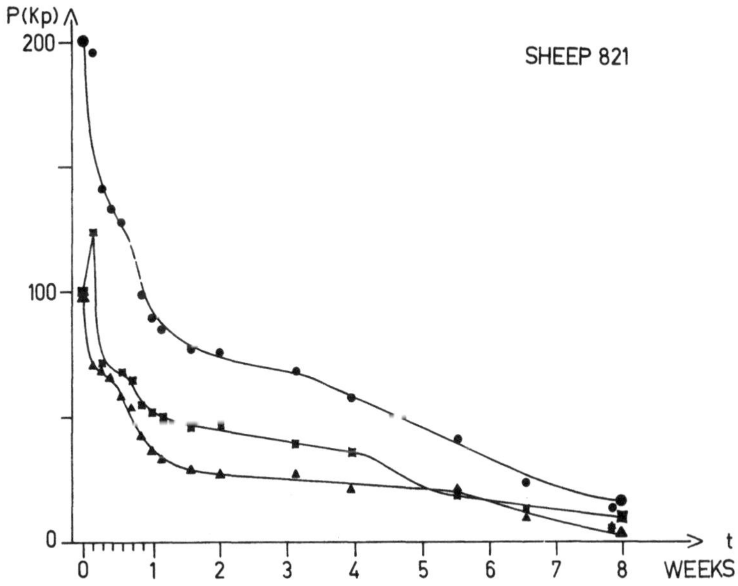

Fig. 25. *In vivo* changes of interfragmentary compression in sheep 821: The axial compression in the two plates shows as an exception a discordant behaviour during the first two days (transposition of pressure?). On the fifth day a new rapid decline in pressure occurs in both plates, perhaps as a result of local overcharge. After the fourth week a last steep reduction in pressure occurs terminating at a final total pressure of only 16 kp

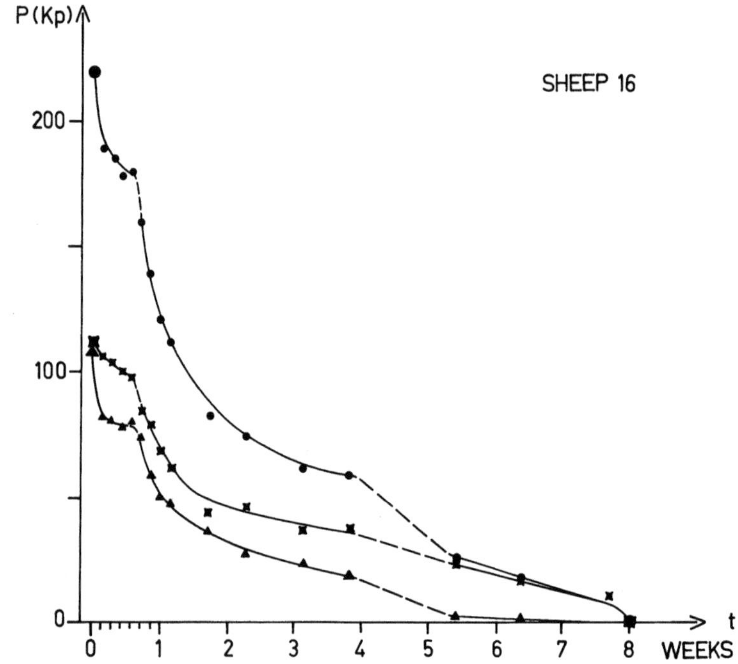

Fig. 26. *In vivo* changes of interfragmentary compression in sheep 16: Biphasic initial pressure reduction with consequent flattening of the pressure curve during the second to fourth weeks. Thereafter, again a more rapid fall-off. In the 4-hole plate compression reaches values around zero towards the end of the fith week, while the pressure in the 6-hole plate reaches zero only after eight weeks

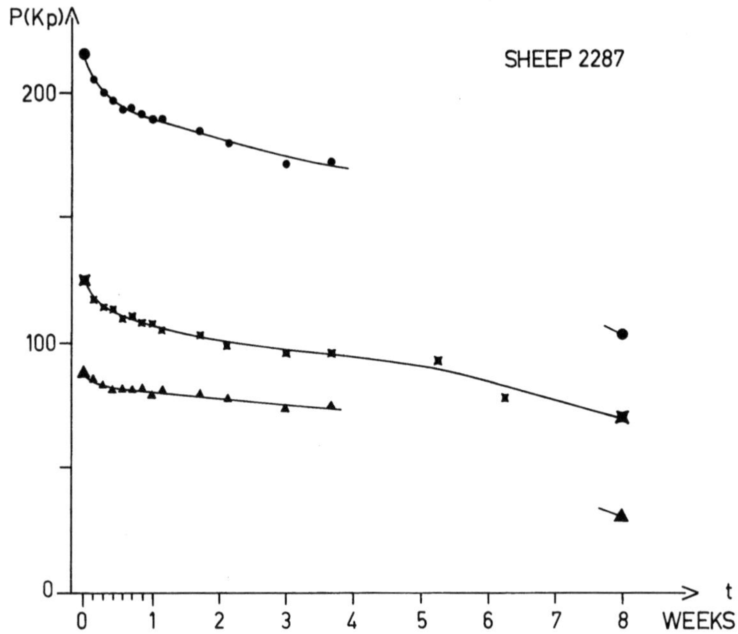

Fig. 27. *In vivo* changes of interfragmentary compression in sheep 2287: After an initial pressure drop and flattening of the curve, the final values indicate a secondary steeper pressure loss also in the 4-hole plate

lowing a break near the gauge chamber, that only a final compression measurement but no final calibration could be performed. In addition continuous measurements were possible throughout the observation period in 11 of the plates mentioned. Due to wire breaks, continuous measurements were no longer possible from the fourth week on in one plate, from the fifth week on in two plates and after the beginning of the eighth week in two plates.

The *in vivo* changes in interfragmentary compression are shown in Figs. 20–27 for each individual plate as well as the sum of both implants. The initial total compression of both plates amounted to 133, 98, 166, 179, 192, 200, 220, 216 kp. In all cases the initial pressure loss was slightly steeper during the first few days and then levelled off. In 6 sheep a secondary steep pressure drop followed towards the end of the experiment. This final reduction was not seen in sheep 741 and 1297. In six out of the eight animals the osteotomy was still under significant compression at termination of the study. In one sheep (16) interfragmentary compression at the end was only slight, and resulted from the force in only one plate. In one sheep (739) both plates had lost their compression. The pressure alterations observed in the two plates of every individual animal paralleled each other after starting from different levels of absolute values. In only one sheep (821) was there an initial pressure loss in one plate, while the force in the other implant increased by the same amount.

3.4. Torque of the Screws

The torque exerted when screws were driven home was measured in 17 of the 19 internal fixations. In the groups "compression with two gauge plates" and "compression with one plate", the values of torque were above 15 cm·kp, usually above 20 cm·kp, for each screw at implantation. In group "no compression with one plate" the torques at implantation varied between 10 and 20 cm·kp [9]. At

[9] The standardised gap of 100 μm between the fragment ends could be maintained during fixation of the plates by alternate tightening and loosening of the screws until all screws were tight. Their individual torque however, often remained somewhat lower than in a compression osteosynthesis. (Biological effects of varying torques are not to be expected [73] and loosening of the screws was not found to be more common, see Table 14.)

Table 14. Maximal torque of loosening of the screws of each side of the plate. Values measured and calculated frequency: The torque required for loosening of the best anchored screw of each side of a plate was measured in all plates. The increments listed on the special screwdriver used for measuring were of the magnitude of 2.5 cm·kp. Values of over 7.5 cm·kp for the torque of loosening were not given in absolute figures since sufficient force transmission is guaranteed above this level. The χ^2-test* was used to determine possible differences between the three groups. The values which were not measured but resulted from calculation are listed in brackets

GROUP	MAX. TORQUE OF LOOSENING (cm.kp) OF EACH SIDE OF THE PLATE					TOTAL
	0.0	2.5	5.0	7.5	>7.5	
"COMPRESSION WITH TWO GAUGE PLATES"	- (0.59)	2 (1.19)	2 (1.78)	3 (5.33)	25 (23.11)	32
"COMPRESSION WITH ONE PLATE"	- (0.19)	- (0.37)	- (0.56)	2 (1.67)	8 (7.22)	10
"NO COMPRESSION WITH ONE PLATE"	1 (0.22)	- (0.44)	1 (0.67)	4 (2.00)	6 (8.67)	12
TOTAL	1	2	3	9	39	54

* $\chi^2=9.8$ when $f=8$. Limits of significance for $p=0.05$: $\chi^2=15.5$. *No difference of statistical significance* occurs between the three groups. This applied also when the values of each classification were compared stepwise in pairs.

explantation the following criteria of "torque of loosening" and "torque of extraction" were used to define a screw which had lost its function by coming loose:

Torque of loosening $\leqq 2.5$ cm·kp
Torque of extraction $= 0$

The implant as a whole was considered to be loose when all screws of one side of the plate fulfilled the criteria listed.

Using these criteria the following results were found in the different groups (see also Table 14):

Group *"compression with two gauge plates"*:
In sheep 739 and 16 the 4-hole plates were loose. All other animals had two solid implants.

Group *"compression with one plate"*:
All plates of these animals were well fixed to the bone.

Group *"no compression with one plate"*:
Only sheep 785 was found to have a loose implant.

3.5. Loading Force

Group *"compression with two gauge plates"*:

The developed force when loading the operated extremity by walking over the electronic platform amounted to 15–30 kp in all eight animals at the end of the experiment. The operated extremities of each animal were fully loaded. Simultaneous registration of the forces through the implanted gauge plates gave the following results:

Sheep: 1297, 878, 15, 821	Significant transmission of the axial forces to both implants. In sheep 1297 the component of force transmitted through the implant was small; most of the strain went through the bone itself (Fig. 28). In sheep 15 the loading force was predominantly directed through the implant (Fig. 29). All these implants continued to produce significant compression.
16	One implant still showed good force transmission, even though it was under little remaining axial compression. The other implant, which was no longer under axial compression, transmitted the axial forces only questionably (Fig. 30).
741, 2287	Good load transmission to one of the two implants; wire break of the other gauge plate. All implants were under significant remaining compression.

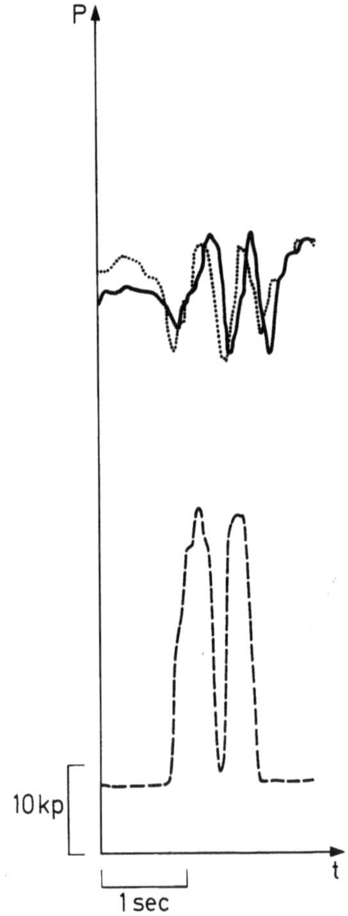

Fig. 28. The loading test in sheep 1297: Only a small component of the loading force (- - -) is transmitted to the 6-hole plate (——) and 4-hole plate (······)

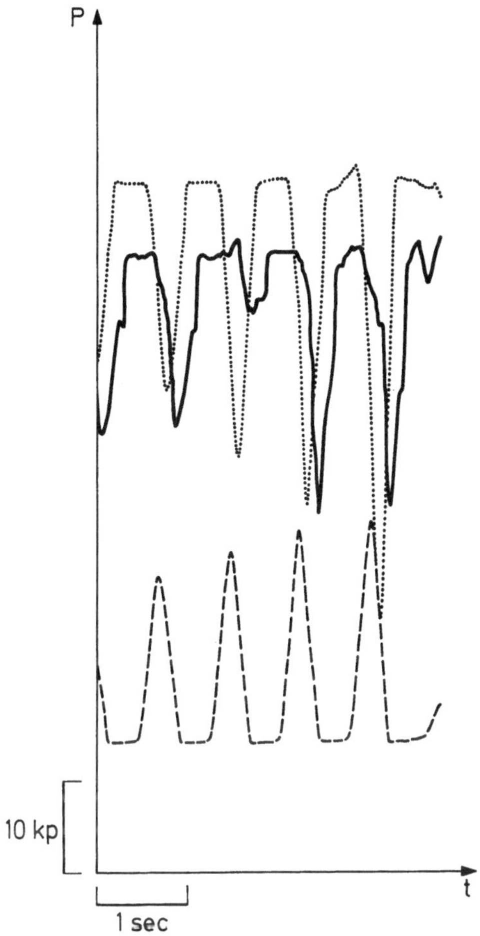

Fig. 29. Loading test in sheep 15: The major constituent of the axial force passes through the 6-hole plate (——) and the 4-hole plate (••••••)

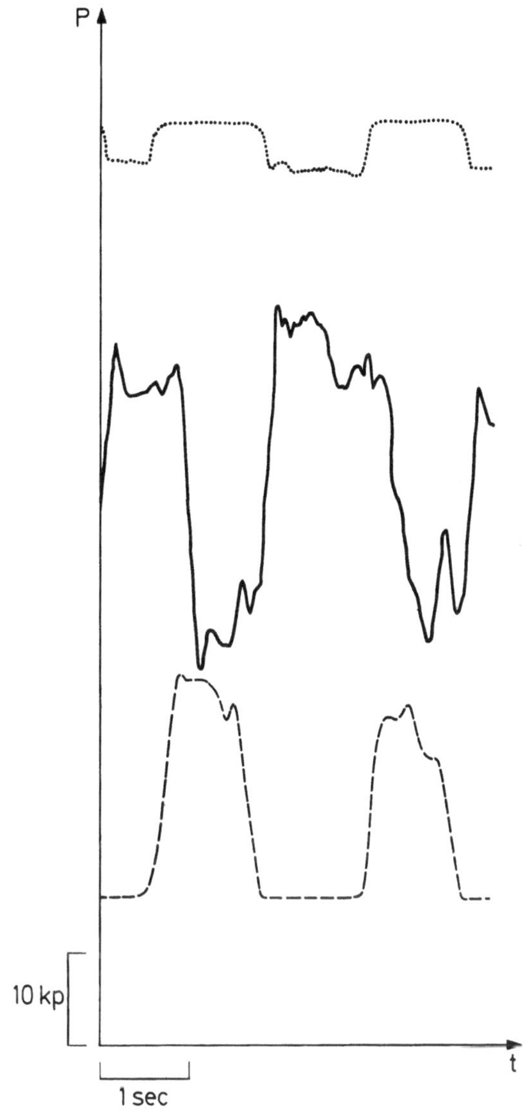

Fig. 30. Loading test in sheep 16: The differences in force transmission to the 6-hole plate (——) and 4-hole plate (•••••) are clearly visible. The (---) line represents the recording from the platform

739 No force transmission to the one plate; no measurement obtained from the other implant due to a wire break. Both implants were no longer under compression (Fig. 31).

Table 15 gives a good review of loading force on the platform, force transmission to the implants and clinical evaluation of loading of the extremity.

Figs. 28–32. Loading force when weighting the operated extremity and force transmission through the implanted gauge plates (loading test): Time is plotted on the abscissa, changes in force on the ordinate. Pressure exerted on the electronic platform and tension stress in the implanted gauge plates led to an upward deviation of the curve. The curve of the loading force ---, the curve of the force through the 6-hole plate —— and the curve of the force through the 4-hole plate •••• (see also p. 13, Fig. 11). Fig. 28 shows the changes in force when the animal walks over the platform, while in Figs. 29–31 the curves are depicted which were obtained from the standing animal with the extremity loaded by induced weight displacement. As a consequence of the rapid changes in induced weight displacement these later curves show the mutual changes in force more clearly (see also p. 13)

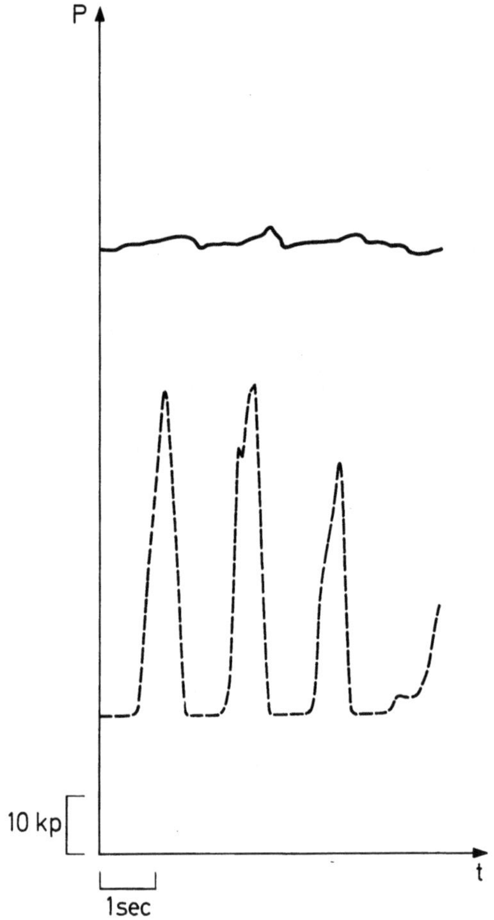

Fig. 31. Loading test in sheep 739: The 6-hole plate (——) registers no force when the extremity is loaded; the wires of the 4-hole plate were broken

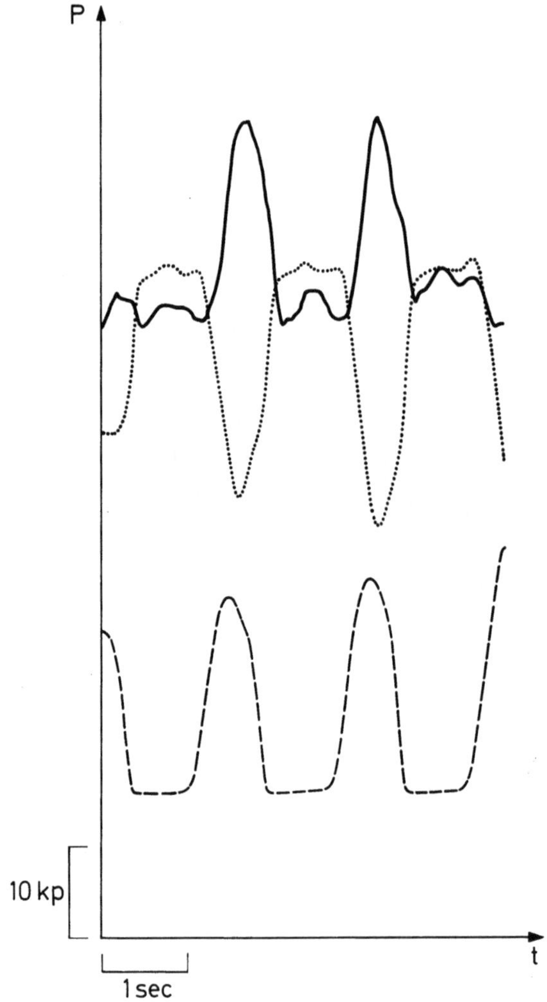

Fig. 32. Simultaneous tension and pressure forces in the two gauge plates implanted in sheep 15: Often sheep 15 showed simultaneous pressure stress on the medial 6-hole plate (——) and tension stress on the posterior 4-hole plate (•••••••) when loading the extremity

When the extremity was loaded, the posterior and medial plates were most often put under tension simultaneously. Only in sheep 15 did this vary so that tension stress on the posterior plate was often associated with compression force on the medial plate, both values of the same order of magnitude (Fig. 32).

Groups *"compression with one plate"* and *"no compression with one plate"*:

Figs. 33 and 34 give the time periods during which the electronic registration of the peak load showed differences of less than 20% in the two hindlegs. The loading of both hindlegs was called symmetrical when the difference was less than 20%, because variations of this magnitude were also found on a repeat of the measurement on the same extremity. Animals in group "compression with one plate" started earlier to fully load the operated extremity. Intermittent interruptions with unweighting were found in both groups. In only two sheep could the uneven load of the hindlegs, as seen on the electronic platform, be recognised clinically.

Table 15. Synopsis of loading force, force transmission to implants and clinical evaluation of loading: Wire breaks were symbolised by WB. The force transmission was classified as follows: + + = Good transmission, > 20 kp; + = Fair transmission, 7–20 kp; (+) = Uncertain transmission, < 7 kp; – – = No transmission

SHEEP	LOADING FORCE ON PLATFORM kp	FORCE TRANSMISSION TO GAUGE PLATE 6-HOLE PLATE	4-HOLE PLATE	CLINICAL EVALUATION OF GAIT
739	20-30	--	WB	1st. and 2nd. week full charge, after 3rd. week frequent alteration between loading and unloading
1297	20-30	+	+	1st. week unloading, after 2nd. week full loading
878	25	++	+	After 1st. week fully loaded
741	20-30	+	WB	1st. and 2nd. week unloading, after 3rd. week fully loaded
15	15-25	+	++	1st. and 2nd. week unloaded, after 3rd. week fully loaded
821	20-25	++	+	After 1st. week fully loaded
16	30	++	(+)	1st. week unloaded, after 2nd. week fully loaded
2287	25	++	WB	1-3 weeks frequent change from loading to unloading. After 4th. week fully loaded.

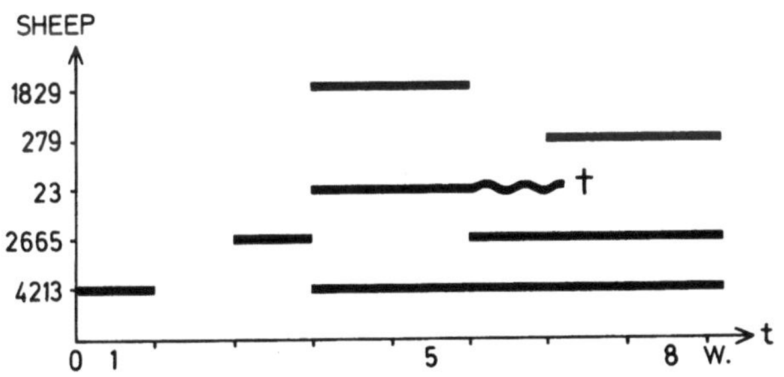

Fig. 33. Schematic plot of the time periods during which the load of both hindlegs was symmetrical (group "compression with one plate"): Full weight bearing as measured with the electronic scale started somewhat earlier in these animals than in group "no compression with one plate" (see Fig. 34). In two sheep full weight bearing was interrupted by temporary non-weight bearing. Sheep 23 suffered from vertigo in the sixth week and was sacrificed one week later

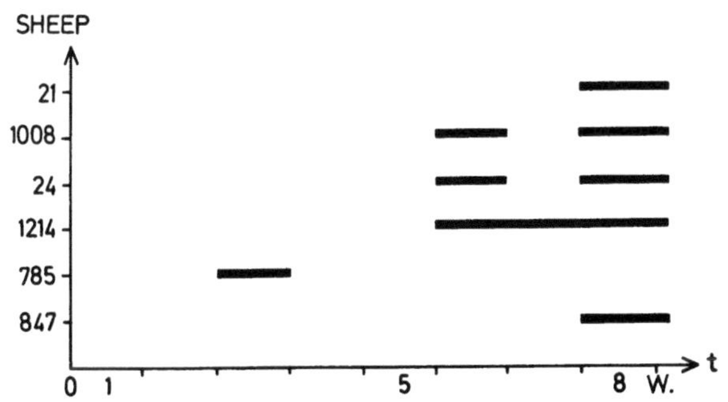

Fig. 34. Schematic plot of the periods of equal charge with both hindlegs (group "no compression with one plate"): Full weight bearing was most commonly started in the sixth week. Three sheep began again to non-weight bear after an initial phase of full weight bearing. By termination of the experiments one sheep had not again fully loaded its operated extremity

3.6. X-Rays: **Plain Films** (Table 16)

The independent evaluations of the X-rays by six different examiners showed good conformity. There existed only minor time-differences in regard to the first appearance of a sign; that is, a finding may have been recognised or described by one examiner only on the X-ray following (two weeks later) the X-ray on which it was initially recognised by the other examiners. The radiologic evaluation of the cases was based on the conventional plain films. The X-ray pictures taken of the explanted bone using the special Faxitron technique (see p. 16) were very rich in contrast. They will be compared with the microradiographic films in Figs. 37–39. The histological aspects of the microradiographic examinations as well as the microangiographic results will be discussed in the chapter on histology (see p. 49).

We will first describe the individual elements of the radiologic changes before summarising the results in the three different groups.

Callus. Borders were often not sharp and the callus itself showed an uneven structural architecture. It was spindle shaped and extended clearly over the osteotomy borders. In all groups the callus was most pronounced on the lateral and, additionally, often on the anterior side of the tibia. It appeared as the first sign of the bony reactions on X-rays of the *third and fifth* week—very seldom later. In those rare cases in which callus was present simultaneously with an osteotomy that appeared united on X-ray, the callus mass decreased in size towards the end of the experimentation period.

Osteolysis. Cortical defects of bone substance were most commonly found simultaneously in the osteotomy zone, around the screws and underneath the plate. They often appeared in the *fifth* week—rarely earlier. On occasion the diagnosis could be made only in the seventh week.

Sequestra. Pieces of cortical bone separated from their surroundings most often lay in large resorption cavities. Extensive sequestration was found in all groups, most commonly however in group "no compression with one plate". This sign usually first appeared on X-rays from the *fifth and seventh* week, and sometimes only in the ninth week.

Sclerosis. This apparent intensification of the bony structure at the fragment ends was most commonly first seen in the *fifth* week. In 3 out of the 16 cases with sclerosis, the diagnosis was made only in the seventh and once only in the ninth week.

Fracture Line. In most cases the fracture line remained clearly visible on X-rays as a wide, sharp line and had not disappeared at the time of termination of the experiments.

A complete fracture union on X-ray, called "complete *healing*" by the clinician, was found in one case only (sheep 4213 of group "compression with one plate") after the eight weeks of observation. We therefore contented ourselves with defining the *pattern* of bony union after eight weeks, without implying that the fracture was completely healed. We distinguish thereby the following patterns of bony union:

- Healing by primary intention: No periosteal instability callus and only minimal fixation callus; no round edges of the fragment ends or osteotomy gaps.
- Healing by secondary intention: Much callus, uneven structure, widening of the osteotomy gap.
- No union: No sign of bony union between the fragments.

Table 16 summarises the results found on the plain films.

The contrast between bony union of the primary versus secondary type on X-ray examination is shown in the two typical series of X-rays of sheep 739 and 2287, both of which belong to the group "compression with two gauge plates" (Figs. 35 and 36).

The X-rays made of the osteotomy zone of the explanted total bone (Faxitron technique) and of the non-decalcified histological slide (microradiography) are placed side by side in Figs. 37–39. The Faxitron pictures made of a bone which is free from soft tissue and implants show the fracture line more sharply than the clinician is accustomed to seeing it. They do however, demonstrate the differences in the healing results exceptionally clearly. The microradiographic pictures help to detect the correlations between X-ray and histology. The results found in the three groups of our experiment are hereby described.

Table 16. Synopsis of the X-ray findings: The evaluation of the X-rays by 3 clinicians and 3 radiologists is summarised. Five criteria thought to be most helpful in clinical diagnosis of osteitis were selected. Extensive findings were symbolised with + + +; absence of symptoms with —. In describing the fracture line these symbols were related to its width

SHEEP	FRACTURE LINE	OSTEOLYSIS	SEQUESTRUM	EXT. CALLUS	SCLEROSIS
739	+++	+++	+	+++	++
1297	+	-	-	+	-
878	++	+++	+++	++	++
741	+	-	-	+	-
15	++	++	-	+	+
821	++	++	++	+	+
16	++	++	+	++	+
2287	+	++	-	-	-
1829	++	++	+++	++	+
279	++	++	+	+	+
23	+	+	-	I	I
2665	+	++	-	++	+
4213	-	++	+	+	+
21	+	+	+	++	+
1008	+	-	-	+	+
24	+	++	+	+++	+
4214	++	+++	++	++	++
785	++	+++	++	+++	+
847	+	+	+	++	+

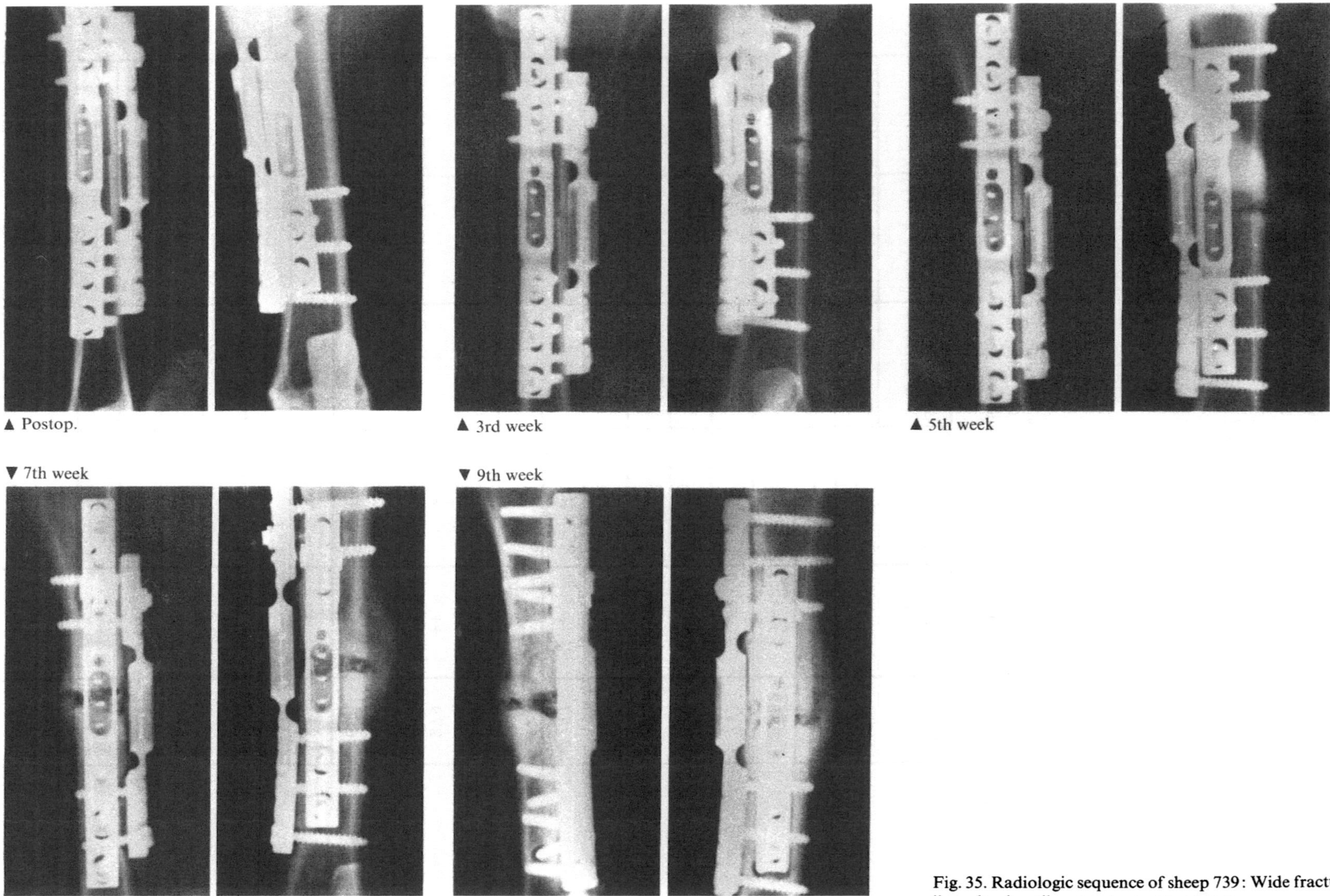

Fig. 35. Radiologic sequence of sheep 739: Wide fracture line, cloudy callus structure, sequestrum

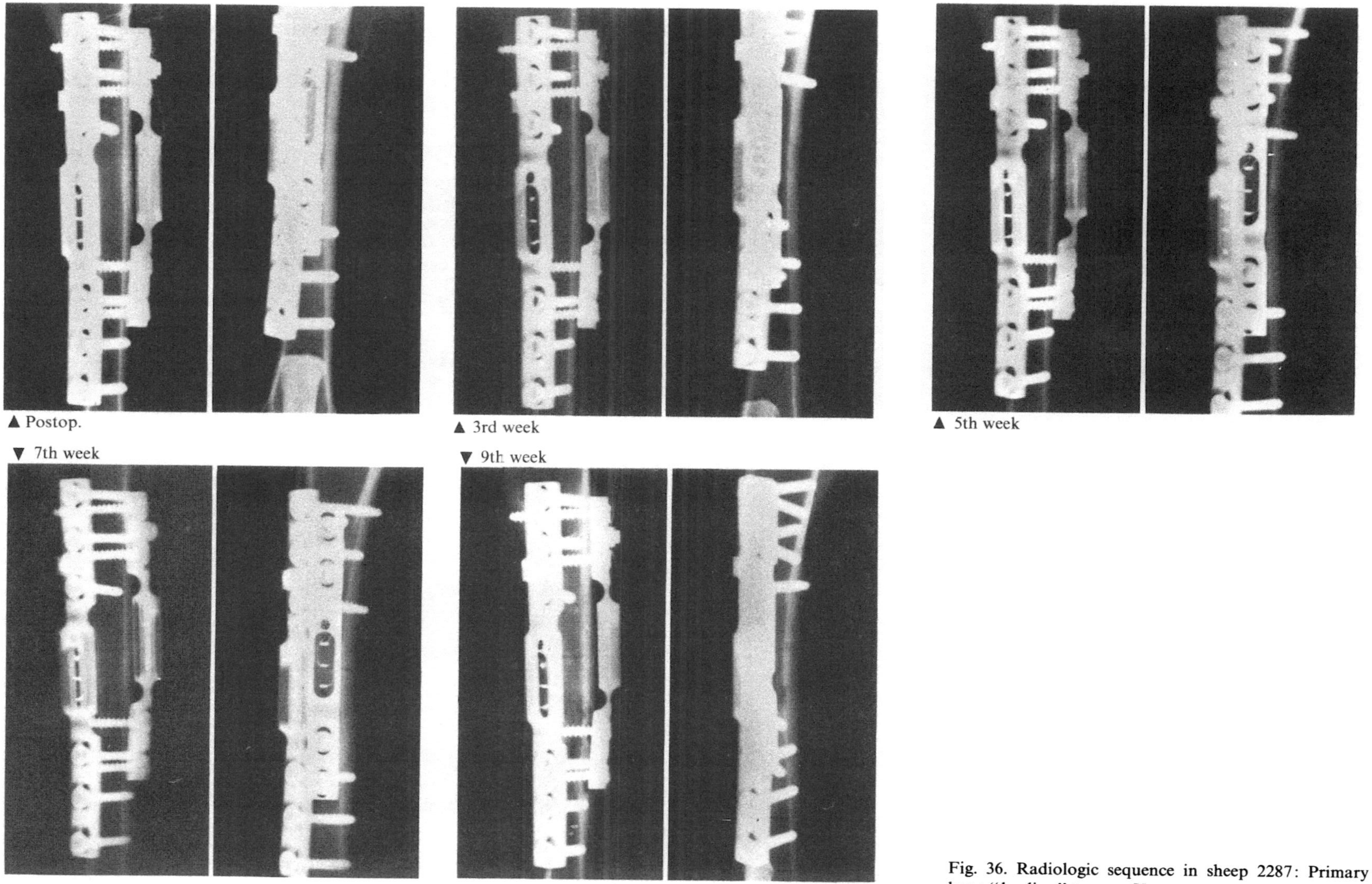

Fig. 36. Radiologic sequence in sheep 2287: Primary bone "healing" type on X-ray

Figs. 37–39. Final radiologic examination (Faxitron and microradiography) of the osteotomy zone: The X-rays taken after removal of the soft tissue and implants show the osteotomy exceptionally clearly. The correlating histological changes are apparent from the adjacent microradiographs. Numbers next to the pictures identify the sheep of group "compression with two gauge plates" in Fig. 37, group "compression with one plate" in Fig. 38 and group "no compression with one plate" in Fig. 39

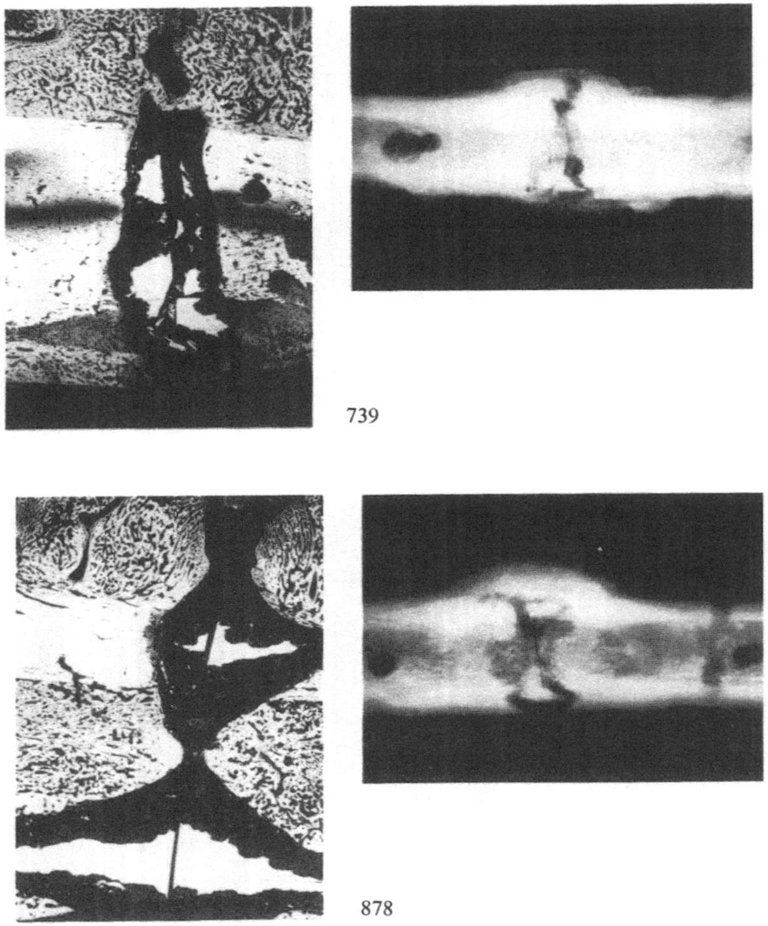

739

878

Fig. 37. "Compression with two gauge plates"

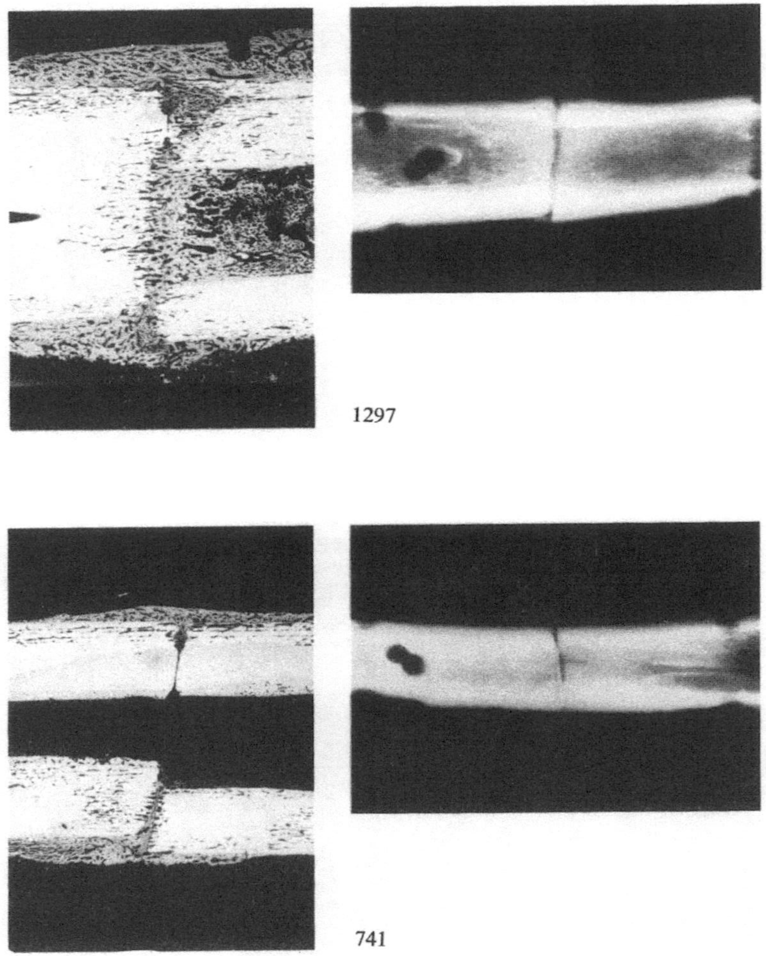

1297

741

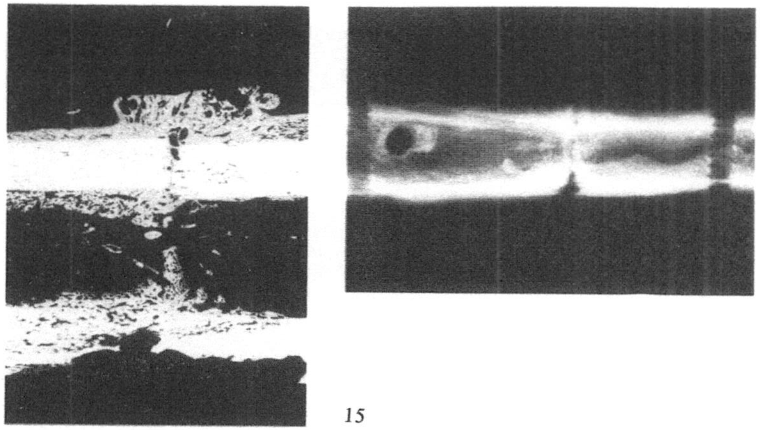

15

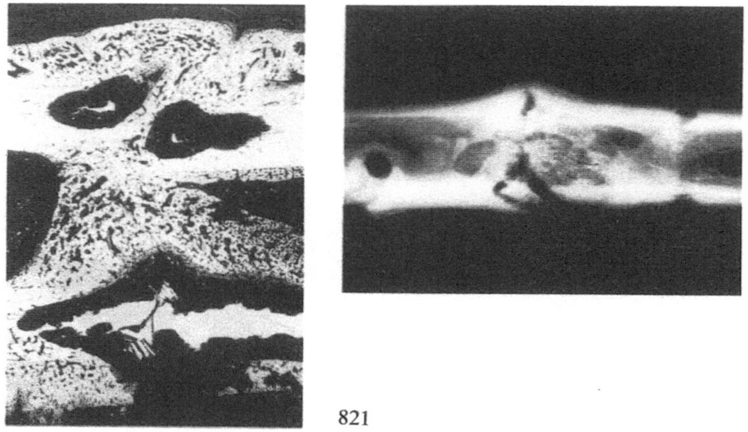

821

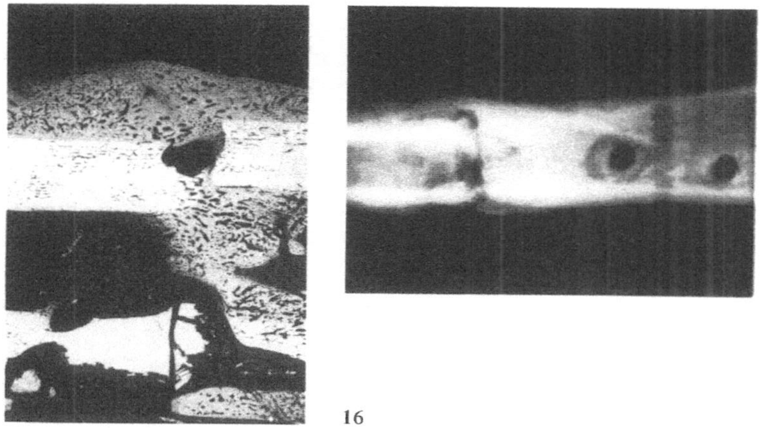

16

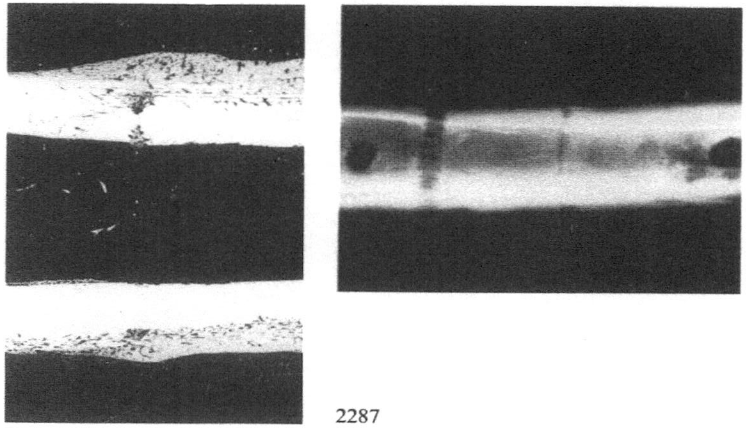

2287

Fig. 37. "Compression with two gauge plates" (continued)

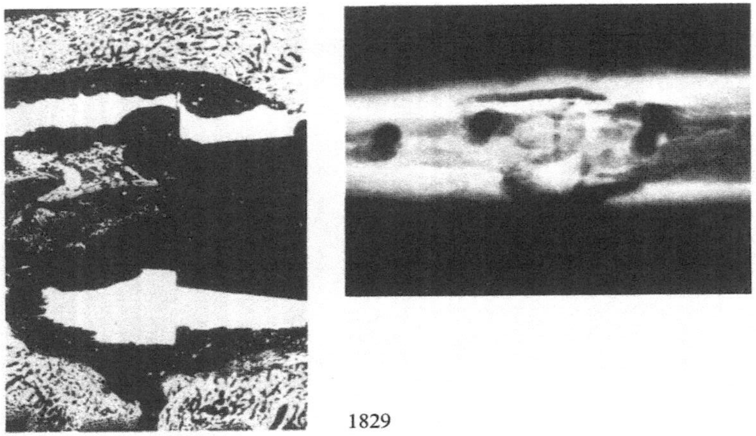

1829

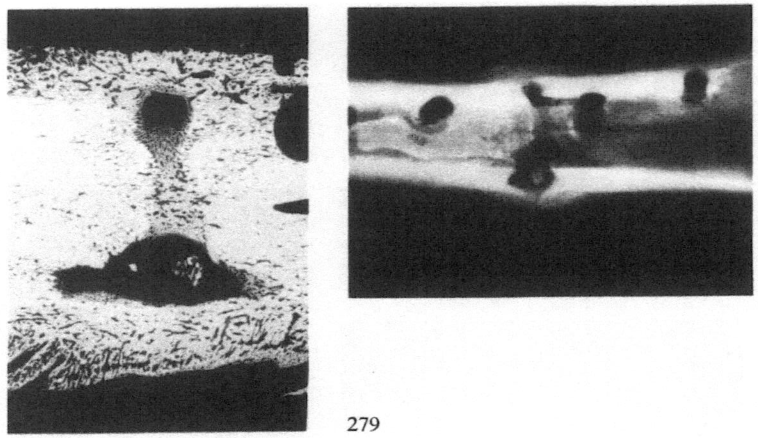

279

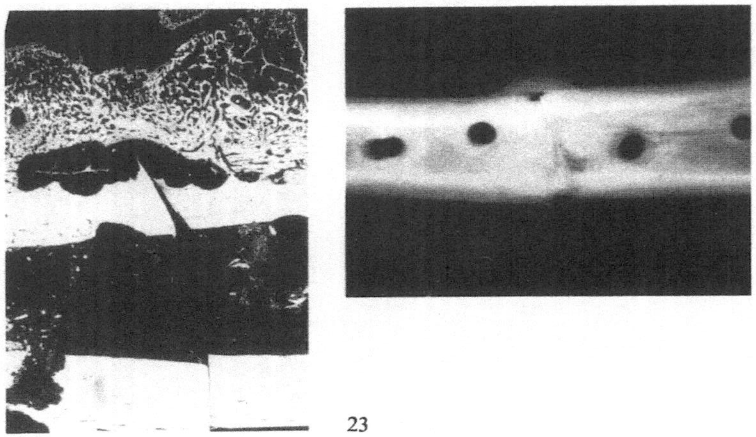

23

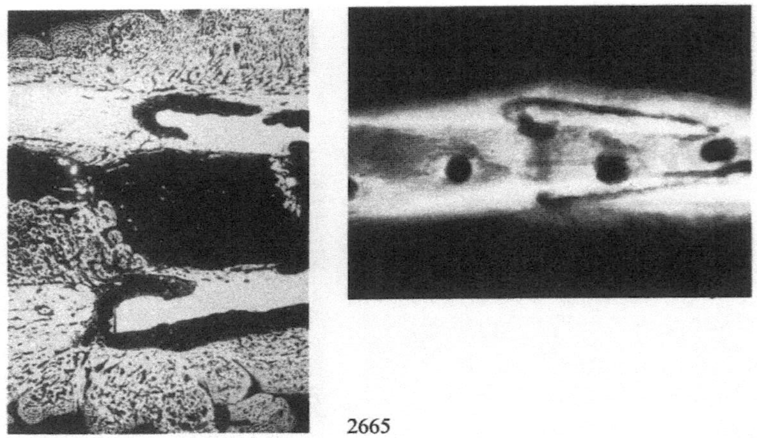

2665

Fig. 38. "Compression with one plate"

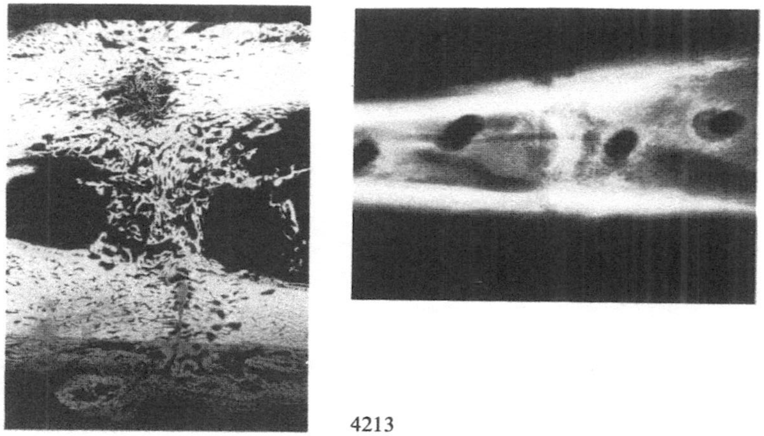

4213

Fig. 38. "Compression with one plate" (continued)

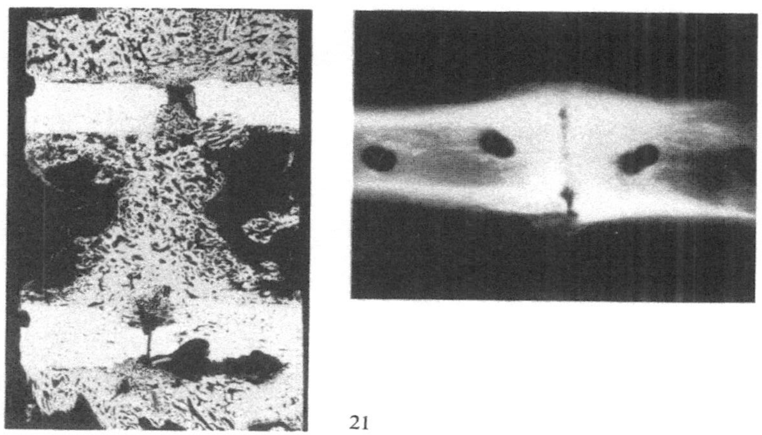

21

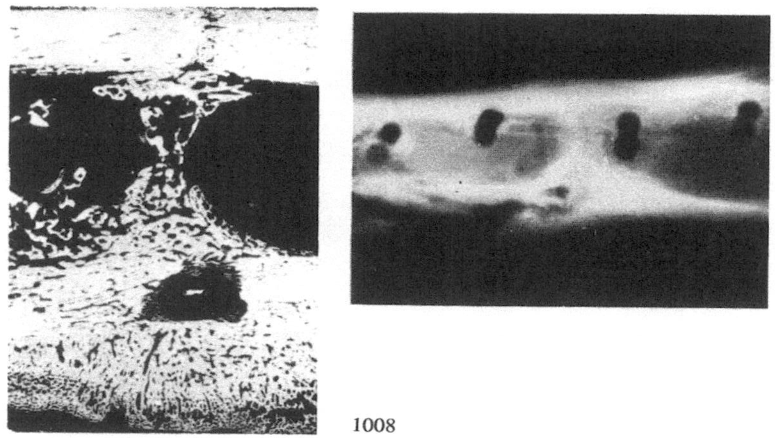

1008

Fig. 39. "No compression with one plate"

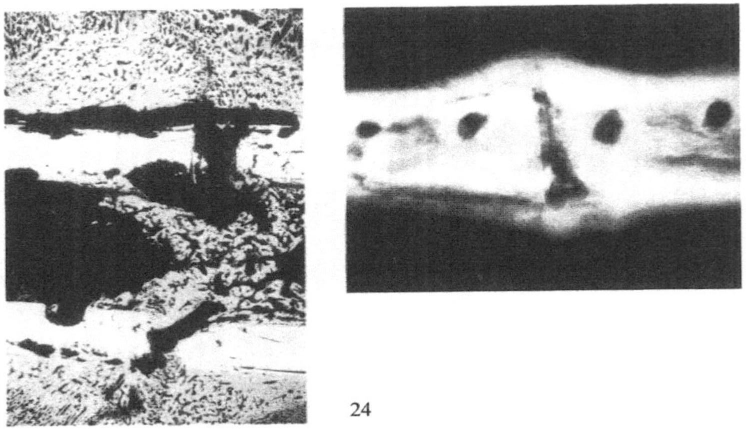

24

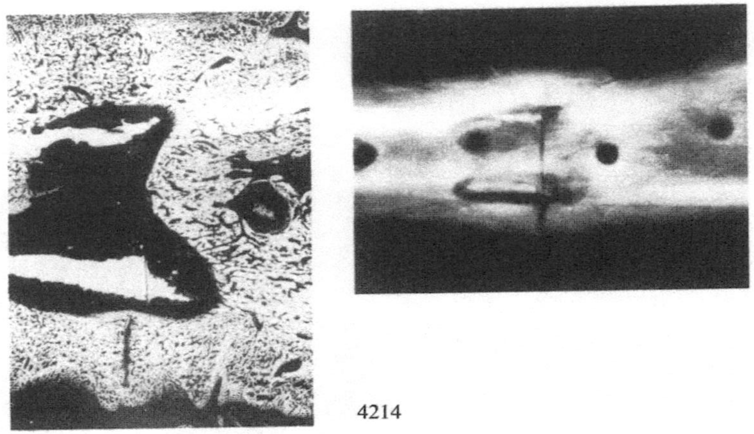

4214

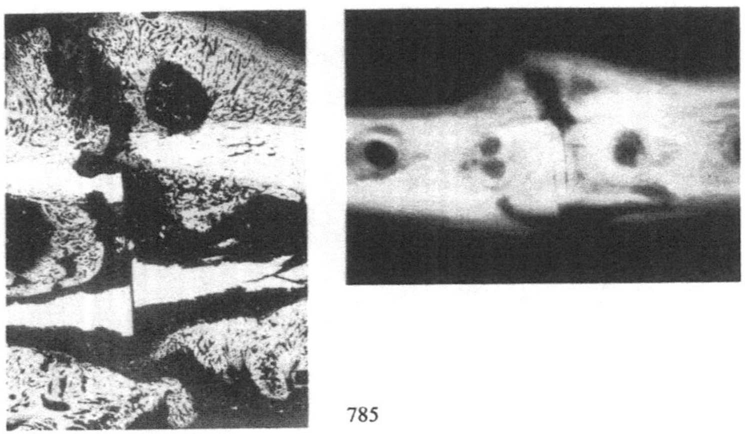

785

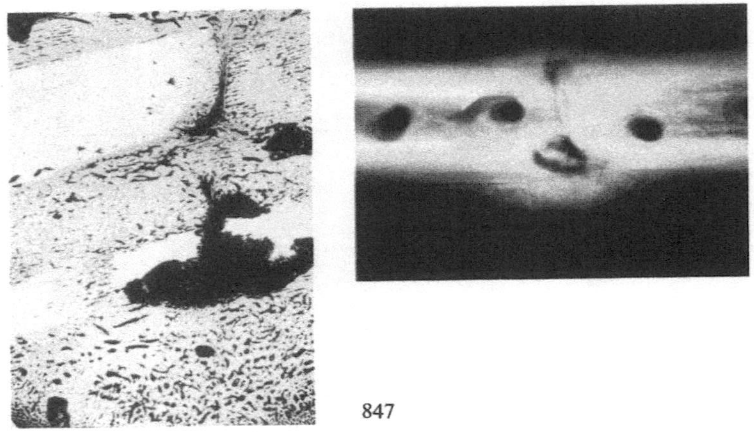

847

Fig. 39. "No compression with one plate" (continued)

Group "compression with two gauge plates":

Sheep 739, 878, 821 and 16 show a secondary healing pattern on X-ray examination (Faxitron). Bony union is uncertain in sheep 739. The adjacent microradiographs are in good agreement with the X-rays except for that of sheep 878, in which there is no bony union seen in this section. Microtome cuts from other locations of the bone circumference show conclusively that bony union by callus apposition has occurred (see index picture of Fig. 42, p. 51). Bony union of the radiologic primary healing type was found in sheep 1297, 741 and 2287 of this group. The microradiographs support this finding. The osteotomy zone of sheep 15 shows some characteristics of primary bone healing, but extensive resorption is present.

Group "compression with one plate":

Only in sheep 4213 can the radiologic characteristics of primary bone healing be found, although the microradiography shows large areas of resorption. The histologic findings on other cuts of this tibia (see *e.g.* the index picture of Fig. 53, p. 56) demonstrate bony union by advanced contact healing. It is however, noteworthy that the osteotomy of this sheep was more proximal than in other animals. All other animals of this group show bony union of the secondary healing type. There is good agreement of the findings seen in the Faxitron pictures with those from the microradiographs.

Group "no compression with one plate":

The sheep of this group show the pattern of secondary bone healing on X-ray examination. In sheep 1008 only one cortex has united; sheep 785 has not bridged the osteotomy at all. The correlation between the two radiologic techniques presented is very good.

3.7. Histological Examination

Common characteristics found at histological examination [10] included: extensive callus formation with bony bridging from one to the other

[10] The different colour sequences were well defined and easily recognised on the histological sections; their colour is, however, difficult to reproduce on paper prints:

alizarin complexone
calcein green
xylenol orange

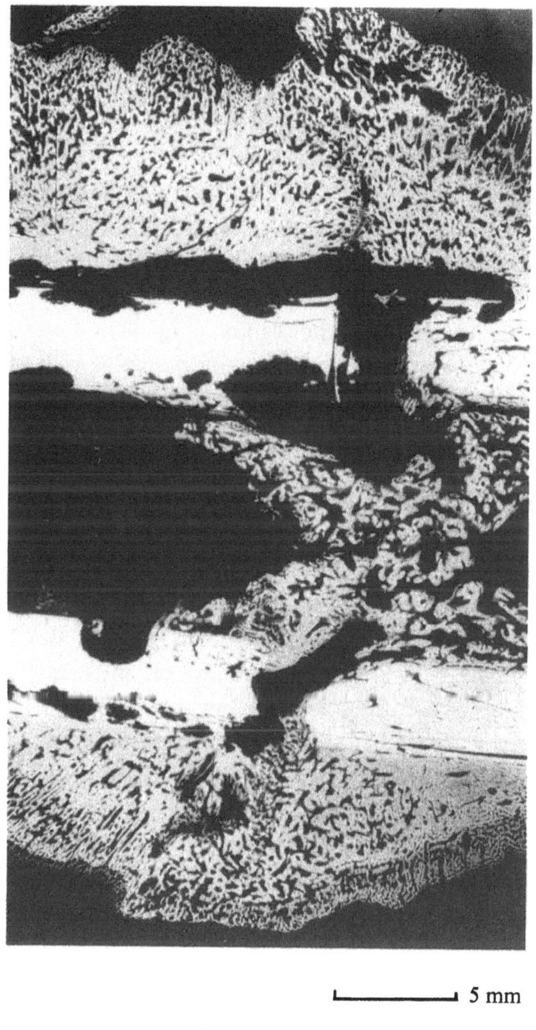

Fig. 40. Microradiographic view of the osteotomy zone in sheep 24 (group "no compression with one plate"): A huge fusiform-shaped callus unites the two main fragments; the endosteal callus formation is less extensive. Severe osteolysis with separation of the callus from the cortex over wide areas

fragment cortex; rarely, bony union of the fragment ends; spreading, local resorption zones of the cortical surface with sequestration; resorption with formation of abscess cavities within the cortex; and finally only slight Haversian remodelling.

We will first discuss the individual histological elements separately and thereafter present the results groupwise.

Callus. Callus formation was, for the most part, extensive. Its bony structure appeared poorly oriented. In most cases the bony union between the main fragments was secured by the appositional callus. In one case only (sheep 785), bridging of the fragments was not complete. Fig. 40 shows a characteristic picture.

On light-microscopic examination, only a few small vessels appeared to be filled with Indian ink. The larger vessels, filled with Micropaque (microangiography) were concentrated in areas where the surface of the cortex was being resorbed underneath the callus (Fig. 41). The deep layers of the callus near the cortex as well as the borders of the spindle-shaped callus mass were rich in vascular supply. Remote from the osteotomy, the callus vessels were oriented predominantly in the longitudinal direction, while they were aligned more in the radial direction in the mid-portion of the callus mass (Fig. 42).

The spindle shape of the periosteal callus, extending well past the osteotomy proximally and distally, was best recognised on microradiographic pictures (see p. 49, Fig. 40). The inner layers were rather dense and appeared non-oriented or, in places, of a radial configuration. The outer layers were more spongy. In many cases a clear orientation in layers was typical in the peripheral zones. The area of final bridging was often clearly visible over the osteotomy. The contact between callus and cortex was planiform and in places the callus was anchored plug-like in the outer cortical layers, best observed on fluorescent microscopic examination (Fig. 43). In the area of the fragment ends the periosteal callus grew into the plane between the fragments (Fig. 44) or retracted recess-like from the fragment ends (see p. 49, Fig. 40). The endosteal

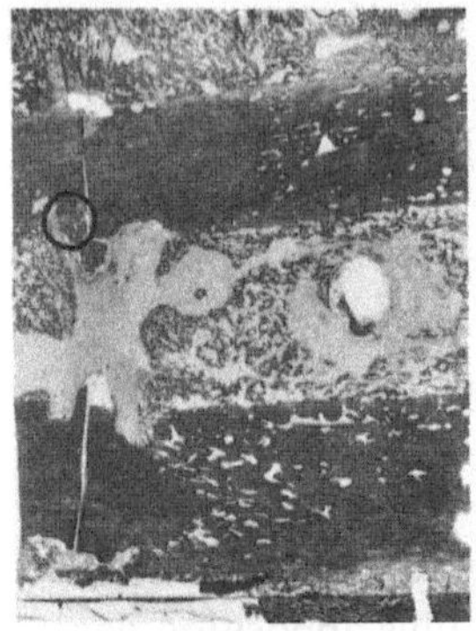
[11]

↓

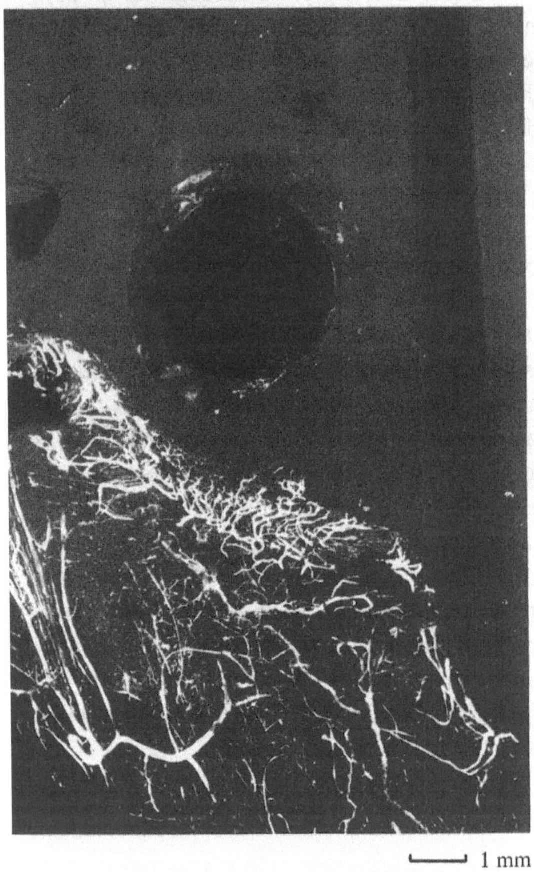

1 mm

Fig. 41. Detail view from a microangiographic picture of sheep 23 (group "compression with one plate"): Strong magnification of a resorption zone shows a dense network of vessels. A completely inactive osteotomy (↓) is recognisable. There is an abscess cavity seen within the cortex near the osteotomy

[11] The index pictures used for orientation were mostly reproductions of microtome sections, which gave us a chance to extend the histological documentation. The small index picture and the main photograph do not however, always correspond exactly as to location and the black circle gives only the approximate location.

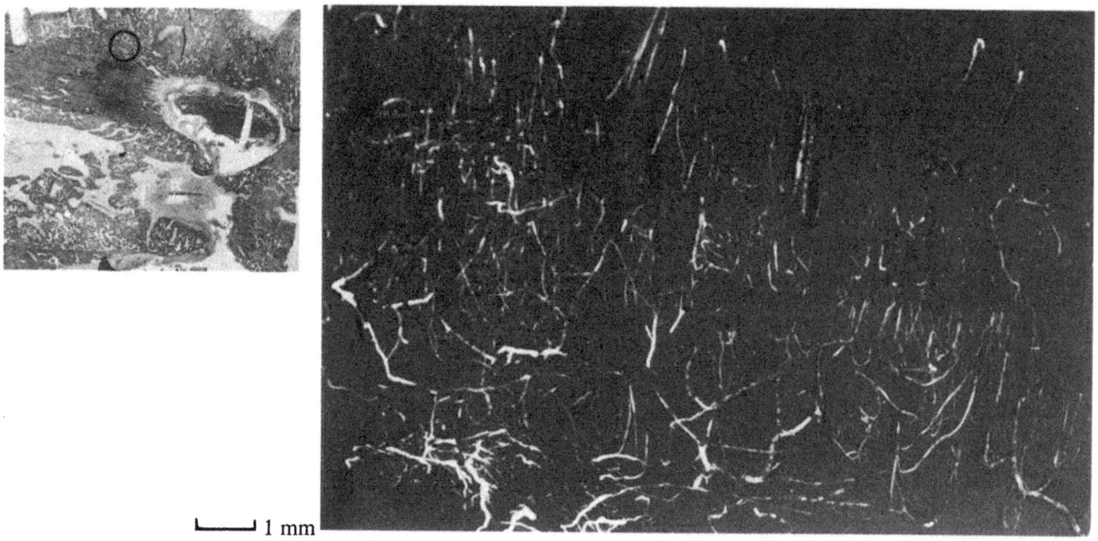

Fig. 42. Detail view from a microangiographic picture of sheep 878 (group "compression with two gauge plates"): On high magnification a more radial orientation is seen in the middle layers of the large callus tumor while near the cortex (lower portion of the picture) the vessels run more longitudinally

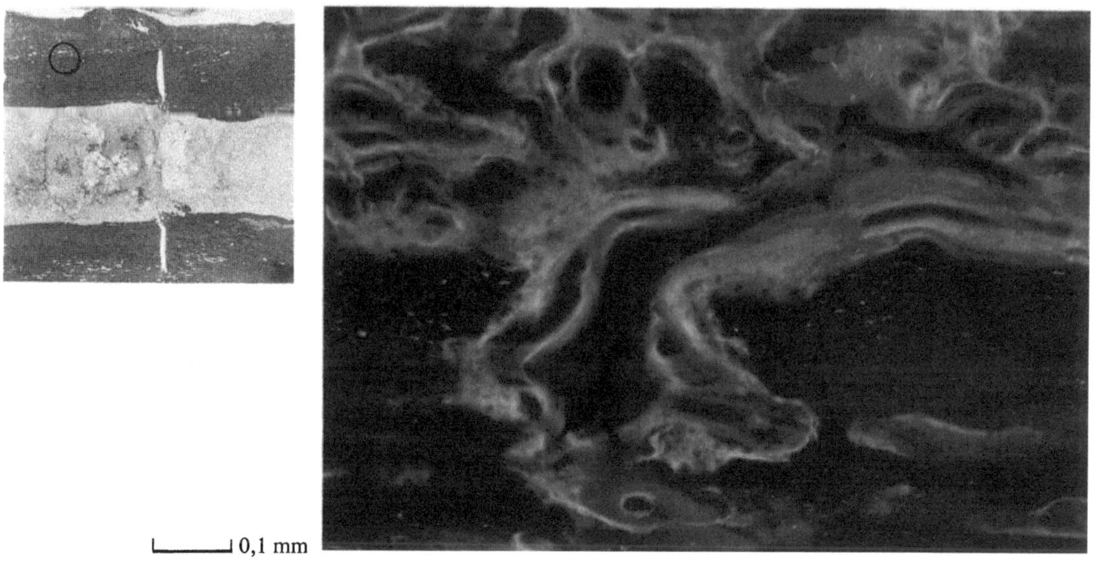

Fig. 43. Anchoring of the periosteal callus in the outer cortex layers: In one place the appositional callus enters the outer cortical layers by plug-like approximation (sheep 2287, group "compression with two gauge plates")

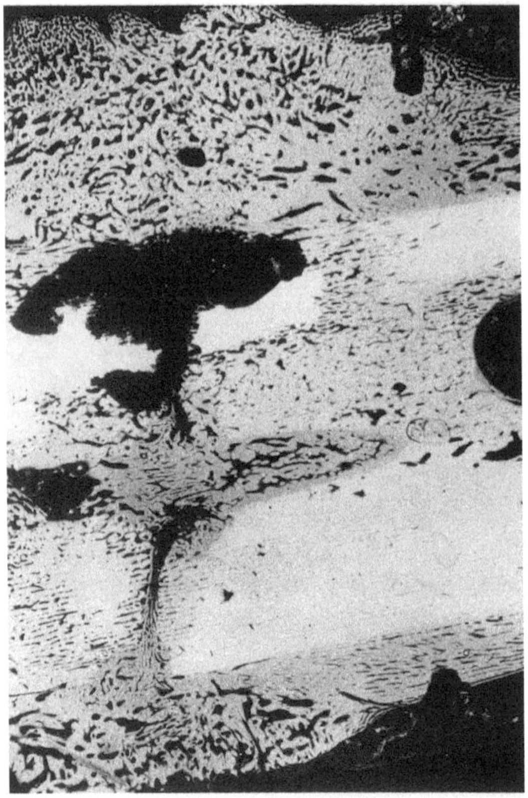

5 mm

Fig. 44. Microradiographic picture of the osteotomy zone in sheep 847 (group "no compression with one plate"): On this longitudinal cut it can be seen that the periosteal callus enters the osteotomy zone between the fragments on one side, while a large resorption cavity is causing a sinus on the opposite side. Note the zones of active remodelling which delineate an incomplete sequestrum

callus was most commonly observed as not very dense and only slightly oriented.

On fluorescent microscopy, calcein blue (second and third week) as well as xylenol orange (fourth week) were deposited mainly in planes within the immature periosteal callus. Calcein green (fifth and sixth week) as well as alizarin complexone (seventh week) appeared in sharp lines in an area of transformation from fibrous to lamellar callus. Often this created the optical effect of colour bands (Fig. 45). The new formation of bone peaked in the fifth to sixth week, but was still active in the outer layers at the end of the experiments. The timing of endosteal callus formation paralleled that of the periosteal changes in most instances.

Resorptive Processes. The cortical bone surfaces were affected by resorptive processes oriented in planes. Bone resorption proceeded from multiple points and caused separation of sequestra.

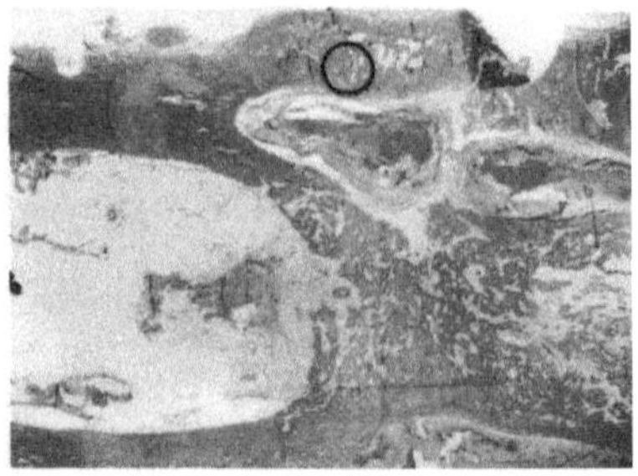

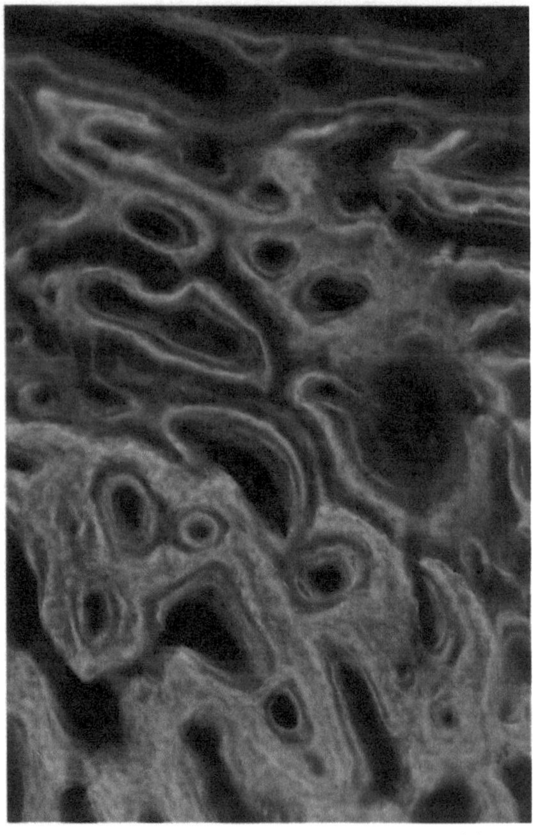

0,1 mm

Fig. 45. Structure of the appositional callus on fluorescent microscopy: Near the cortex the labels given in the fourth and fifth weeks (orange = Xylenol orange, green = calcein $green_1$) were deposited in planes, while the labels of the sixth and seventh week (green = calcein $green_2$, red-brown = alizarin complexone) marked the transformation of fibrous to lamellar bone (sheep 821, group "compression with two gauge plates")

Fig. 46. Spherical erosions with formation of a sequestrum (sheep 16, group "compression with two gauge plates"): Microradiography showing spherical erosions, which may lead to sequestrum formation when proceeding simultaneously from periosteum and endosteum

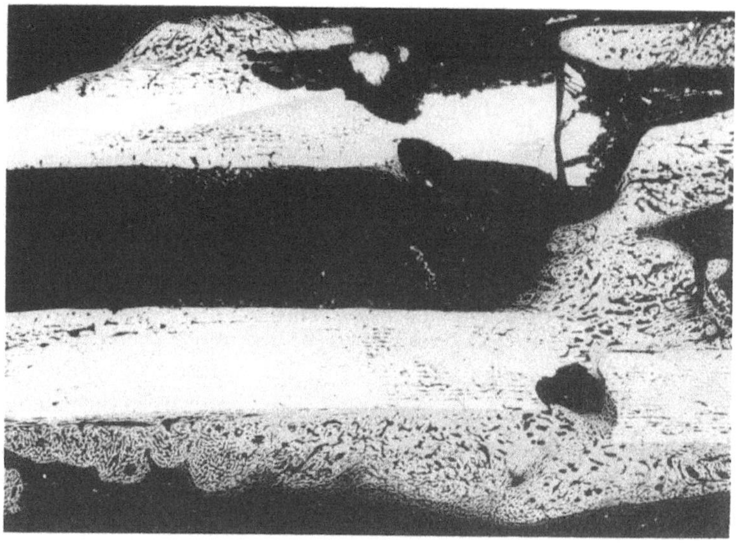

5 mm

Within the cortex resorption cavities were found filled with abundant round cells.

In the light microscopy examination, vessels filled with Indian ink entered the resorption fronts from tissue adjacent to the bone. In some areas spherical erosion fronts were seen (Fig. 46). The resulting cavities were often crossed by fine branching vascular arborisations (Fig. 47). The sequence of resorptive processes shows simultaneous advancement of the erosions from periosteal and endosteal sites, with resulting release of a sequestrum (Fig. 46). Often the entire osteotomy zone was cut out *en bloc,* the osteotomy remaining clearly visible within the sequestrum (Fig. 48). The osteotomy as such was remarkably seldom attacked by the osteoly-

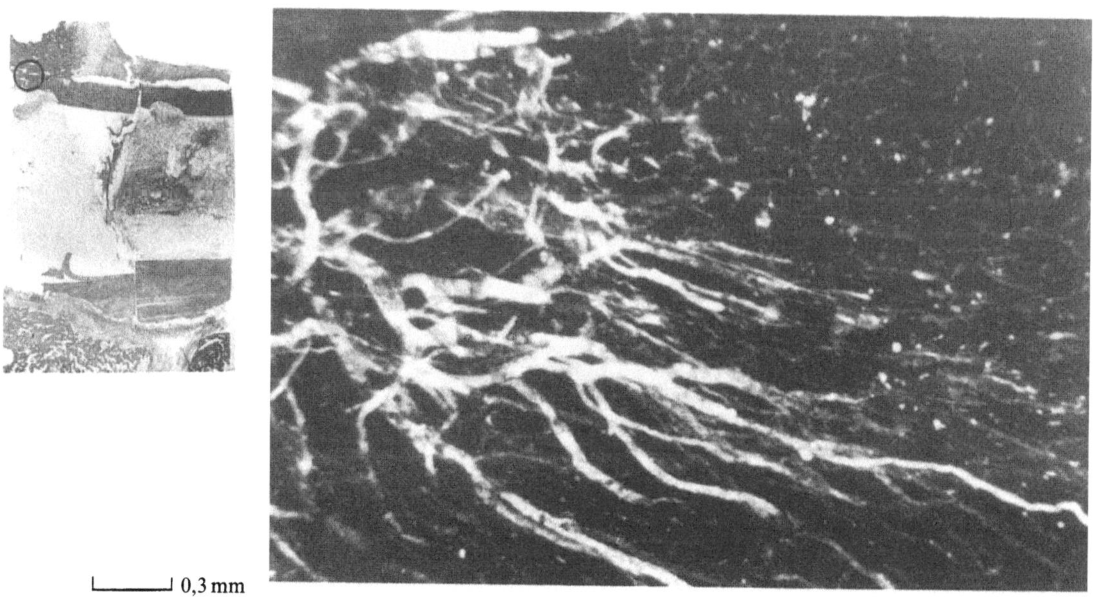

0,3 mm

Fig. 47. Vascular tree in resorption cavity: Often resorption cavities contained a dense vascular network. High magnification of the cavity from the osteotomy zone (from microangiography of sheep 1829, group "compression with one plate")

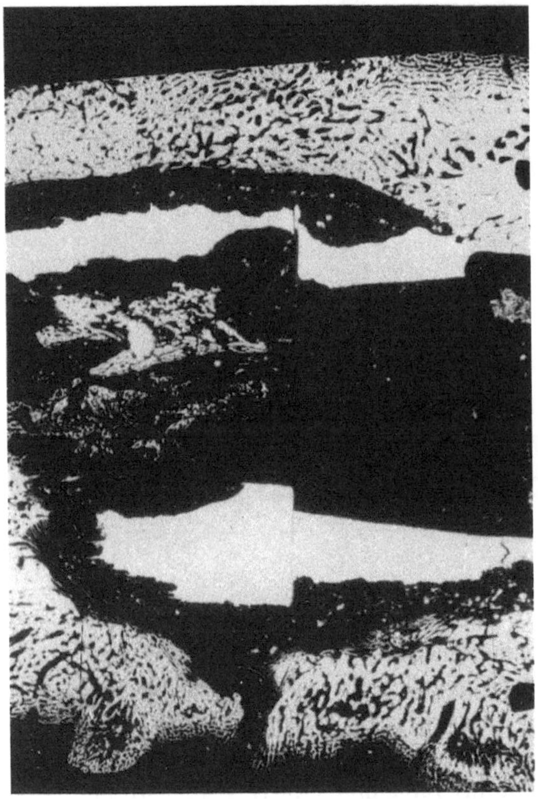

5 mm

◁ Fig. 48. Sequestration of osteotomy zone in sheep 1829 (group "compression with one plate"): The microradiography shows practically full sequestration of the osteotomy zone. The osteotomy itself is barely affected by the osteolytic processes and in only one of the cortices

tic processes. The isolated sequestra were eroded only from their other surfaces exhibiting the aspect of typical resorption fronts (Fig. 49), but not from the osteotomy site. Margins composed of osteoblasts were rare, and new bone deposition was exceptional on these surfaces. A timing of the resorptive processes was difficult, since these resorption fronts rarely ever contained fluorochrome deposits. The few labels encountered indicated that resorption occurred predominantly after the fifth week. The sequestra themselves rarely ever showed bony remodelling and, as a rule, contained no vessels. Bead-like resorptions ("goccie di cera") [29] were not infrequently active in the outer part of the osteotomy plane, reducing the shaft diameter significantly. This type of resorption was found also

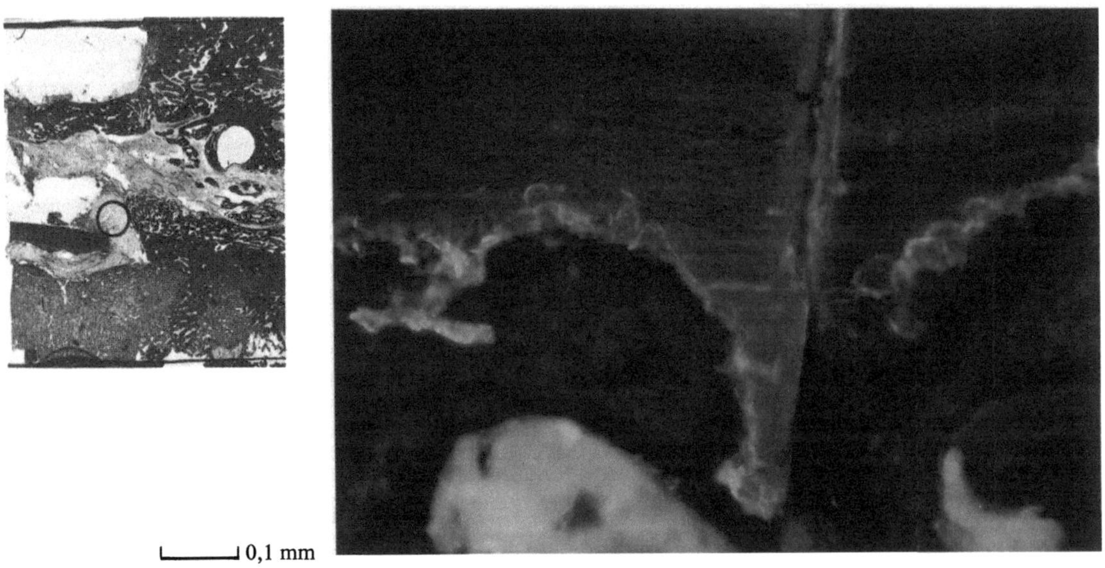

0,1 mm

Fig. 49. Fluorescent microscopy in sheep 4214 (group "no compression with one plate"). Resorptive fronts of sequestrum: Typical fronts of resorption labelled with calcein green and alizarin complexone (fifth to seventh week). The osteotomy itself is not attacked

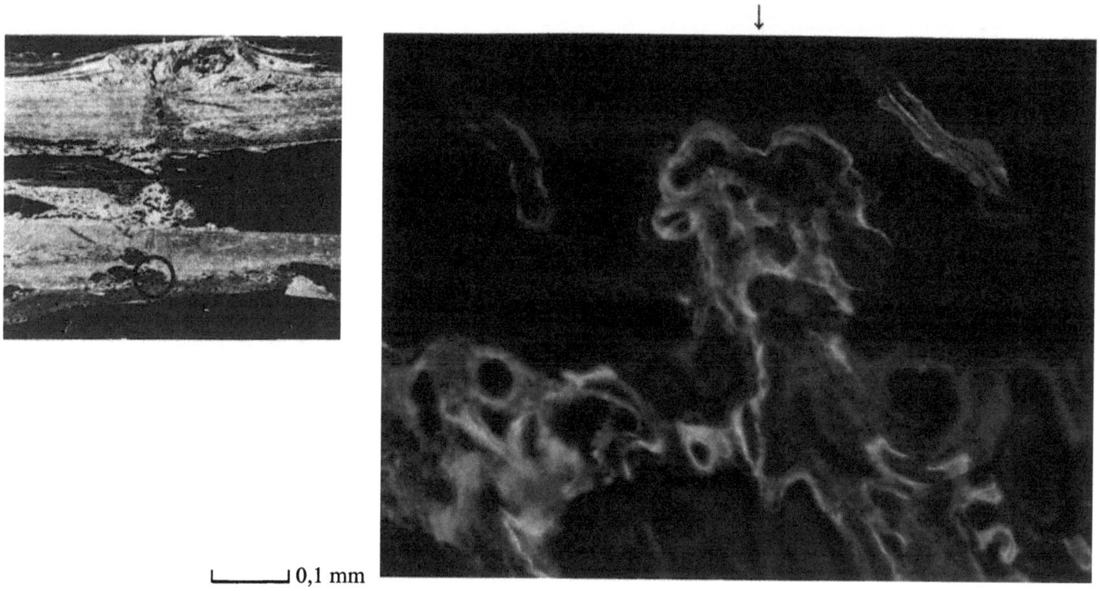

Fig. 50. "Goccia di cera" in the osteotomy zone: The circumscribed resorption cavity is filled with lamellar bone in the seventh week (red-brown = alizarin complexone). The osteotomy (↓) is barely visible on this fluorescent microscopy picture (sheep 15, group "compression with two gauge plates")

in one case where both cortices were seen, on longitudinal cuts, to contain many areas with contact healing and therefore a circumferential contact of the fragment ends was assumed. These bead-like grooves were later filled with lamellar bone and served then as elements of bony bridging (Fig. 50, and see p. 52, Fig. 44). The resorptive processes attacked the callus often in the vicinity of the osteotomy. Small bone tissue fragments which carried labels were present, as was a simultaneous demonstration of irregular margins of the callus, these two findings together indicating that a bridge, which had most likely originally been attached to both fragment ends, was later separated by osteolysis from the sequestra formed (Fig. 51, and see p. 49, Fig. 40).

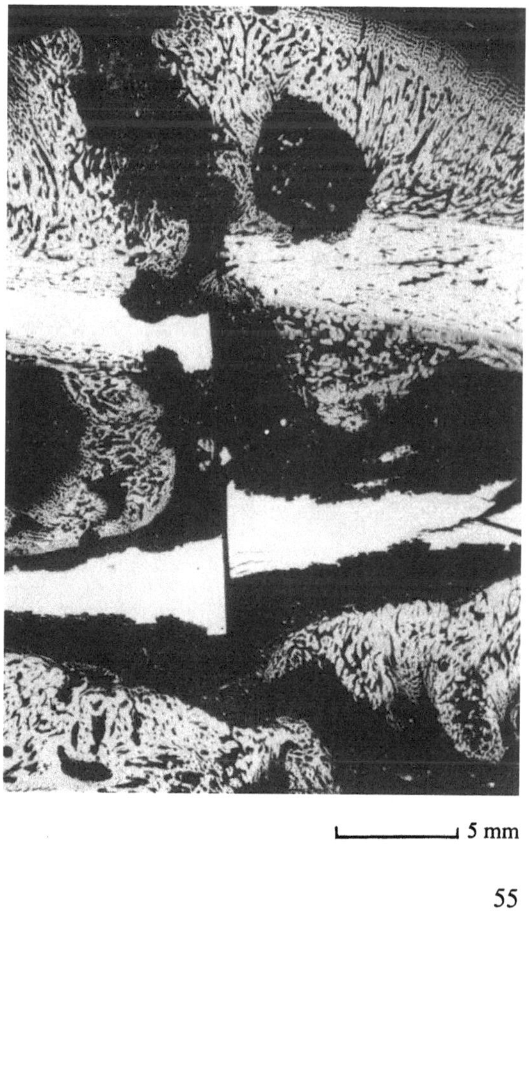

Fig. 51. Microradiography of the osteotomy zone in sheep ▷ 785 (group "no compression with one plate"): The appositional callus formation shows incomplete bridging and no attachment to the sequestra

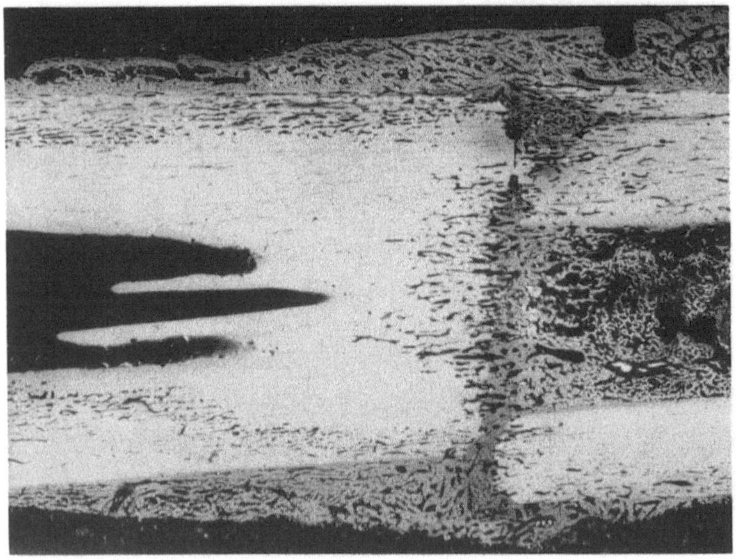

Fig. 52. Zone of contact healing between the main fragments with "goccia di cera", gap healing and Haversian remodelling bands: The zones of Haversian remodelling traversed the cortex in bands leading from the outer to the inner layers. Microradiography of sheep 1297 (group "compression with two gauge plates"). The cut surface runs slightly obliquely which makes the medullary cavity appear on only part of the surface

5 mm

Cortical Remodelling. The remodelling of cortical bone was minor in the bone segments examined. Osteons of longitudinal orientation, often accumulated in oblique bands, were noted crossing the cortex (Fig. 52). Round cells were not encountered in these zones, and osteocytes were clearly visible (Fig. 53). Directly adjacent to the osteotomy, remodelling was often increased with irregular distribution over the fragment ends (Fig. 54). As mentioned, no Haversian remodelling was found within the sequstra (Fig. 55). Only exceptionally did one observe localised remodelling zones within the sequestra. Apposition of callus was found regularly on such

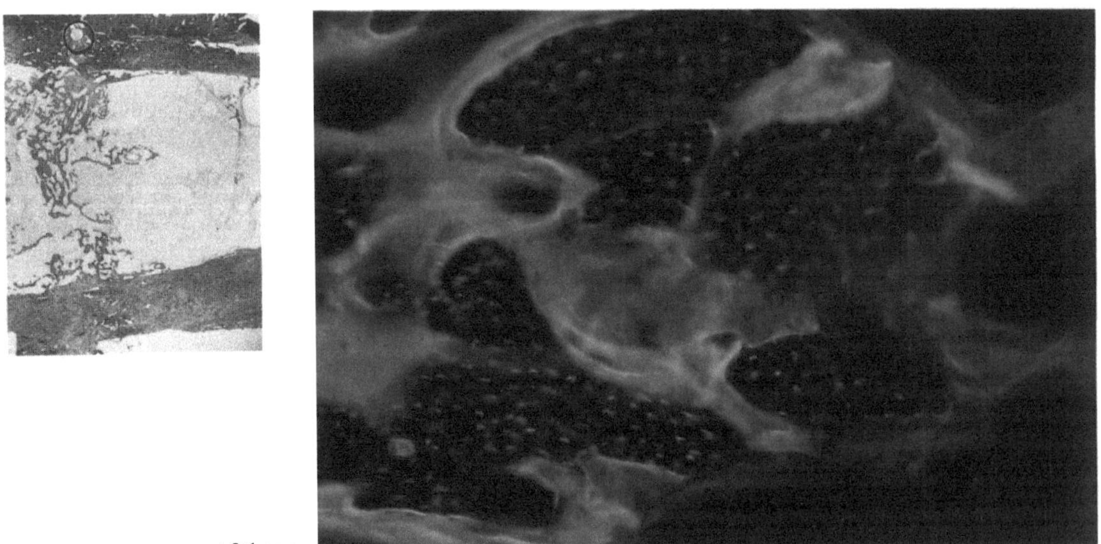

0,1 mm

Fig. 53. Remodelling zone with labelled osteocytes: Deposition of calcein green in (cavities of) osteocytes, which are accompanied by labelled bone deposits in planes (sheep 4213, group "compression with one plate")

sequestra, which were separated from an area of intensive remodelling. The highest rate of remodelling occurred during the fifth and sixth week and was somewhat less extensive at termination of the experiments (Fig. 56).

Comparative microangiographic examination of the vascular tree in the three groups reveal no differences. No correlation was found either between vascular density and type of bone healing, or the extent of osteolytic processes. This was true for the cortex as well as the callus and medullary cavity.

Bony Union between the Fragment Ends. Bony union between the fragment ends was rarely far advanced. Where present it occurred by filling of the osteotomy gaps with fibrous or lamellar bone ("gap healing") [30] or by direct crossing over the osteotomy planes of osteons ("contact healing") [99] when the fragment ends were found to be well adapted[12]. No cortical union was found if the fracture gap was very wide due to osteolysis and sequestration. In such cases bone deposition on the fracture ends was very

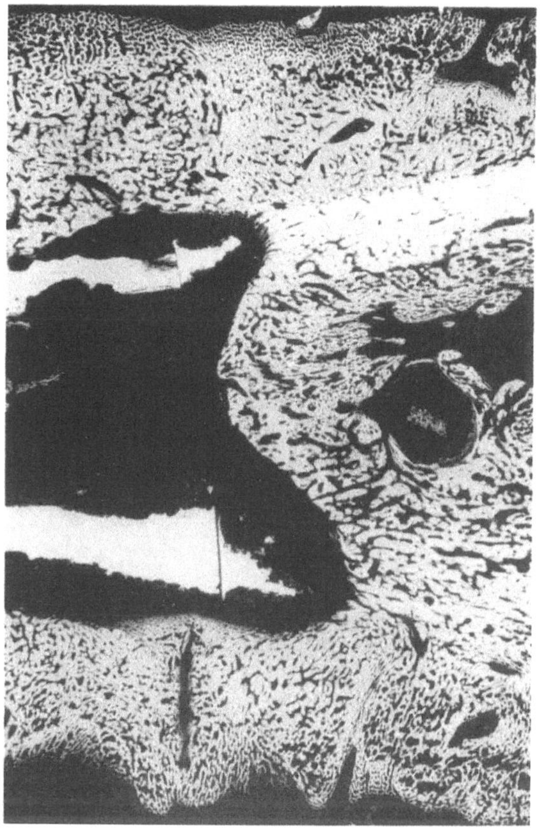

Fig. 55. Microradiography of sequestrated osteotomy zone in sheep 4214 (group "no compression with one plate"): Within the sequestra little remodelling activity is found, while the fragment ends show very active cortical remodelling. The callus in the lower part of the picture shows incomplete bridging

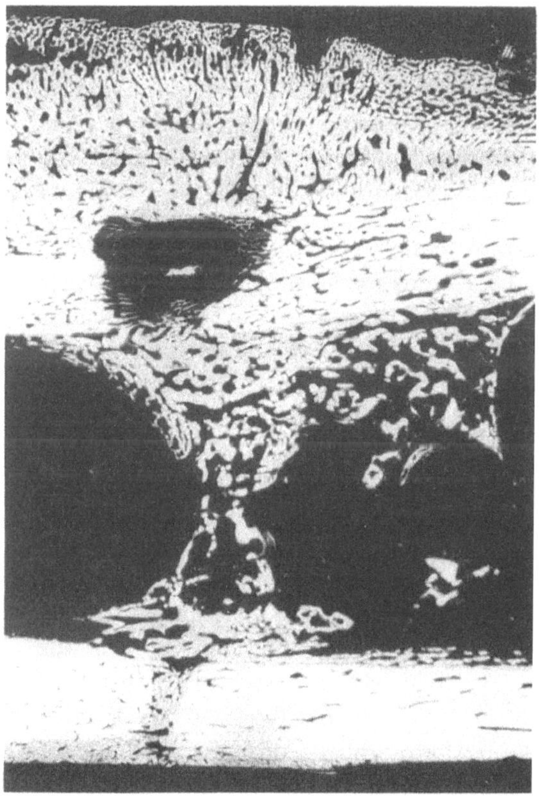

Fig. 54. Haversian remodelling in vicinity of osteotomy zone: Near the resorption cavity increased remodelling activity is found; in the opposite cortex gap healing with little callus (sheep 1008, group "no compression with one plate")

[12] The terms "gap healing" and "contact healing" are used in this communication to describe the *pattern* of bony union on the histological section. No real "healing" as such, in the sense of full restoration or "complete healing" as clinicians refer to it, can be expected to occur within this short interval of 8 weeks.

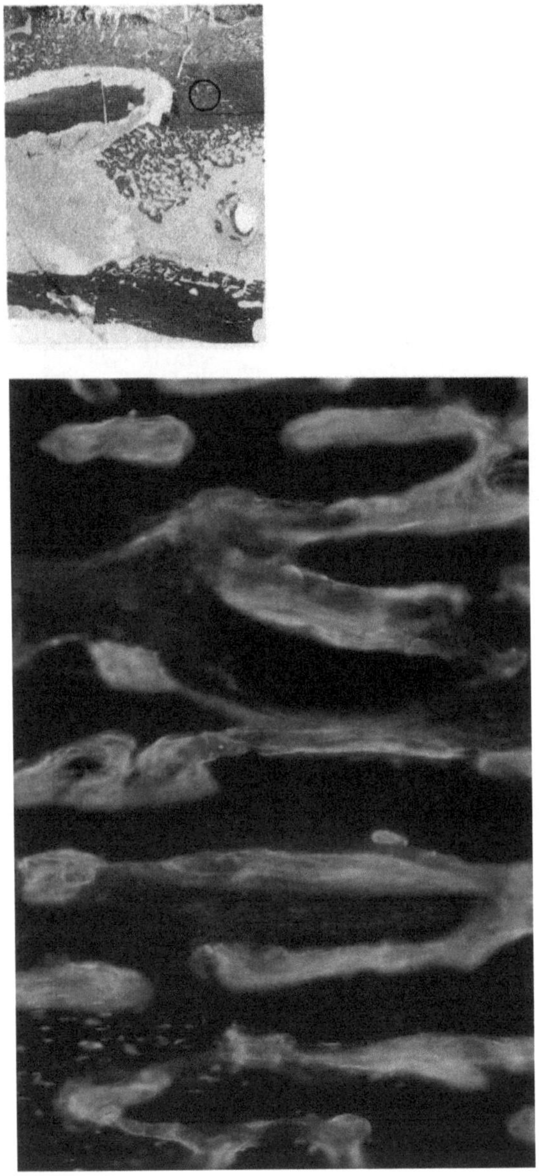

0,1 mm

Fig. 56. Haversian remodelling in sheep 2665 (group "compression with one plate"): Maximal remodelling activity was found in most cases during the fifth and sixth week

little and occurred late towards the end of the experiments (Fig. 57).

Contact healing: On rare occasions osteons reached the osteotomy accompanied by vessels filled with ink; even more seldom they crossed the osteotomy (Fig. 58). The osteons were oriented longitudinally and usually located within the bands of remodelling. No inflammatory cells were found near the osteons. Contact healing most often started in the seventh and eighth week, but at times was already present in the fifth and sixth week.

Gap healing: In the gaps between the fragment ends, which were practically free of round cells, vessels filled with contrast media were found (Fig. 59). Lamellar bone filling the spaces was oriented transversely and was formed independently of the remodelling of bone within the cortex. This can best be seen on microradiographic studies (see p. 52, Fig. 44). In the fifth and seventh week, filling of the gaps was most active (Fig. 60). In a few cases intracortical osteons had begun to cross these gaps in the longitudinal direction towards the end of the experiments (Fig. 61).

We shall henceforth examine each sheep in each group separately with respect to the histological changes previously described. Before this, however, it should be noted that a finding common to all animals was the presence of bone abscesses of differing extent throughout the entire cross section.

Group "compression with two gauge plates": The characteristics of *primary bone healing*[13] were present in five animals. Most frequently contact healing of one cortex was present with simultaneous gap healing on the opposite side of the bone circumference.

Sheep:

2287	Contact healing of both cortices on longitudinal cuts. Only slight resorption. Minimal callus formation.
1297, 15	In one cortex the elements of gap healing are seen; on the opposite side characteristics of contact healing with or without "goccie di cera". Resorptive processes of minor extent yet causing an intracortical cavity on the side with contact healing in sheep 15 (Fig. 62). Little callus formation.

[13] See footnote on p. 57.

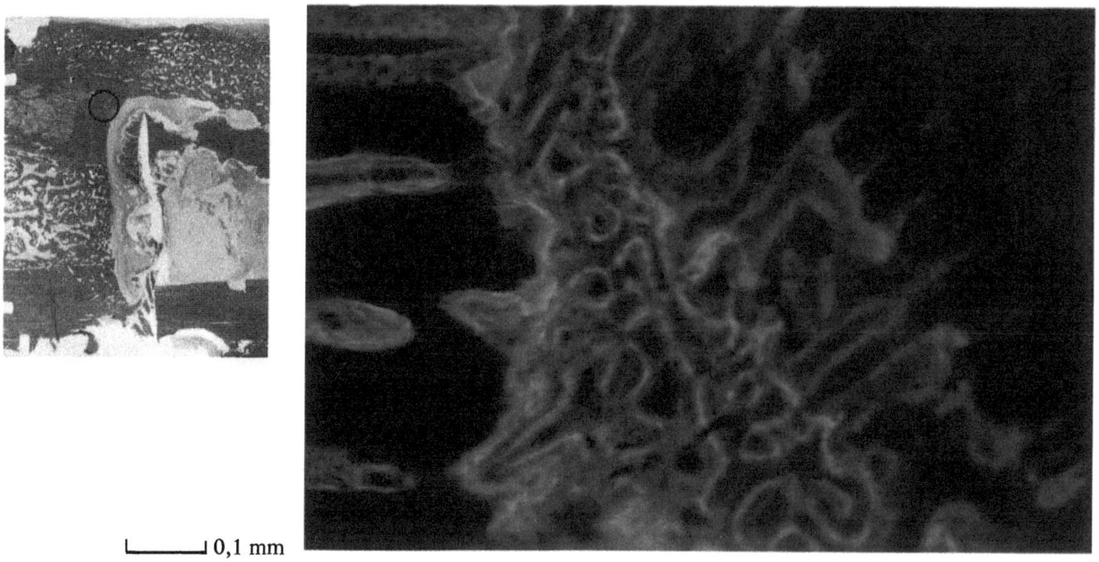

Fig. 57. New bone formation around osteolytic focus: Deposition of new bone on fragment ends occurred predominantly in the eighth week (red-brown = alizarin complexone, emerald-green = no label). Fluorescent picture of sheep 16 (group "compression with two gauge plates")

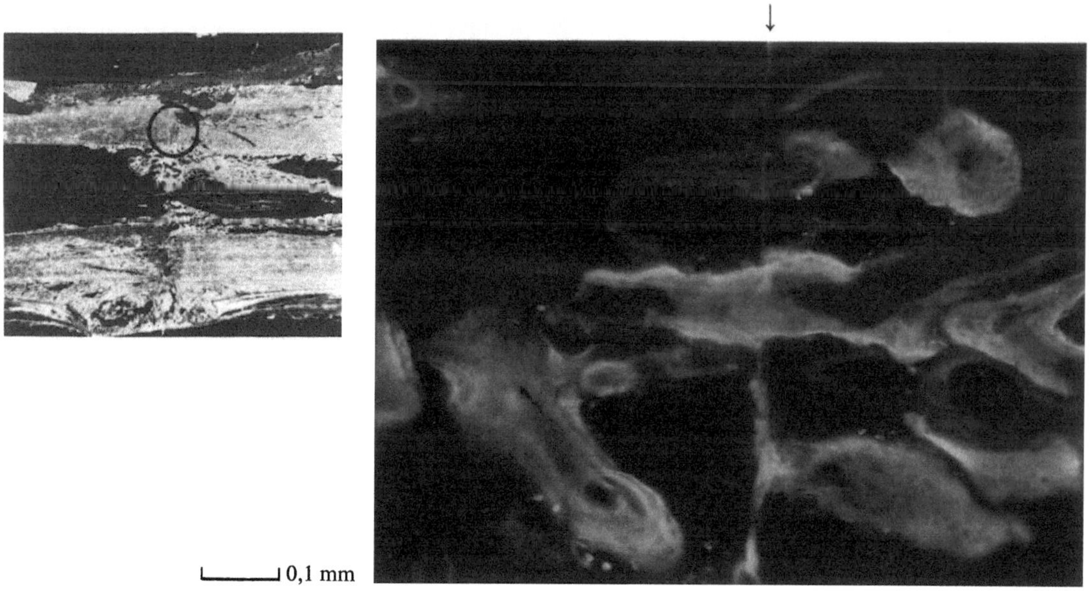

Fig. 58. Contact healing of an infected osteotomy on a sheep tibia: A few osteons cross the osteotomy (↓) of the tibia after the fourth week (sheep 15, group "compression with two gauge plates")

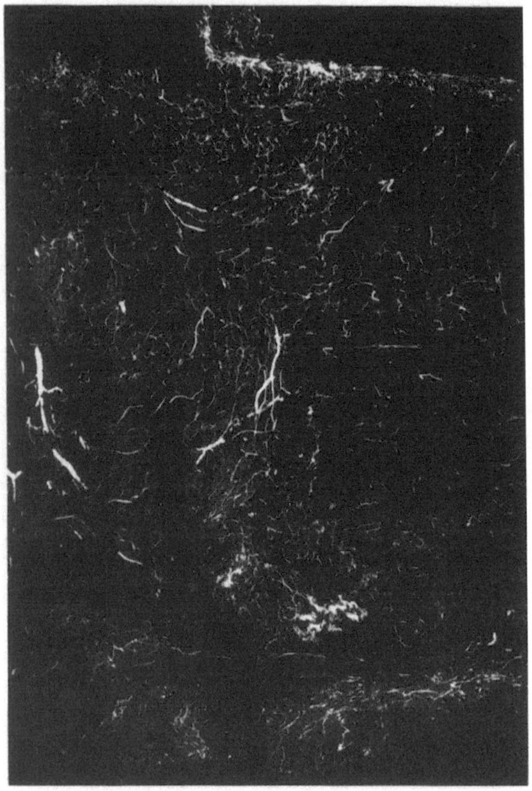

3 mm

Fig. 59. Microangiography of an osteotomy zone with gap healing: In between the two fragment ends, cut tangentially and united by gap healing, a dense vascular network is found (sheep 1297, group "compression with two gauge plates")

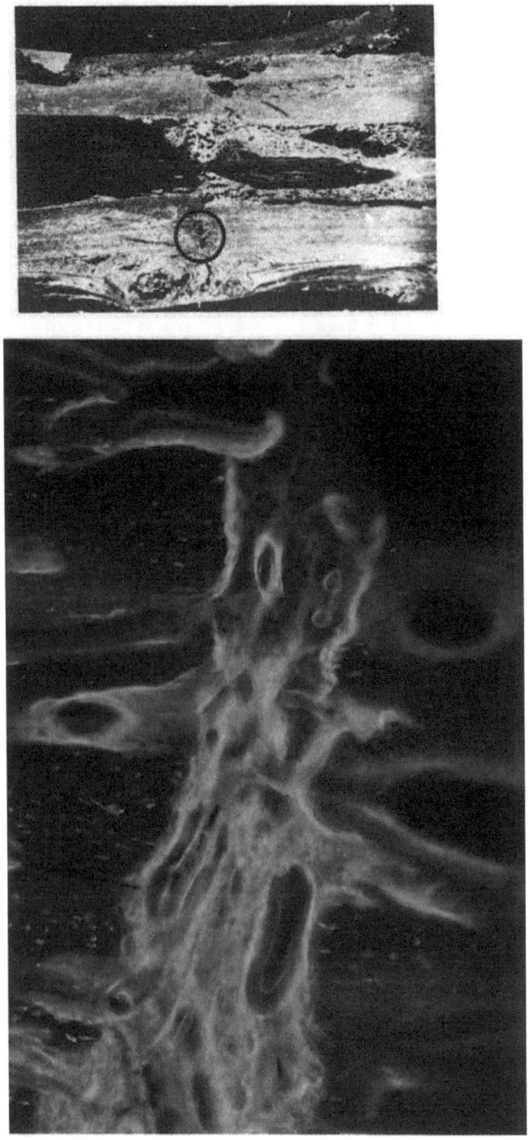

0,1 mm

Fig. 60. Gap healing of the infected osteotomy of a sheep: In the fifth and sixth week the gap between the fragment ends was filled with lamellar bone oriented in transverse direction. From this gap, filled with new bone, osteons started to grow into the cortex in a longitudinal direction (so-called "plugging"), (sheep 15, group "compression with two gauge plates")

741 On one side of the cortex gap healing which began late in the course of the experiment. On the opposite side signs of bony union are barely recognisable. Little resorption or callus formation.

821 On one side of the cortex union with characteristics of gap healing; near the osteotomy, resorption cavities. On the opposite side extensive sequestration of the entire osteotomy[14] covered by incomplete callus bridging. Endosteal union of the fragment ends by callus.

Therefore, this case will not be classified as union of the mary type of bone healing.

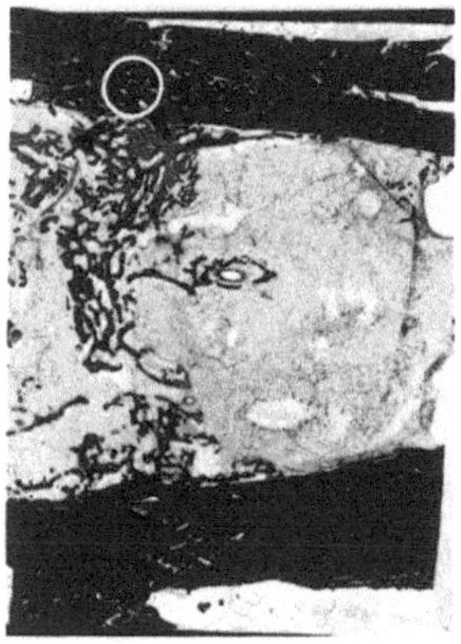

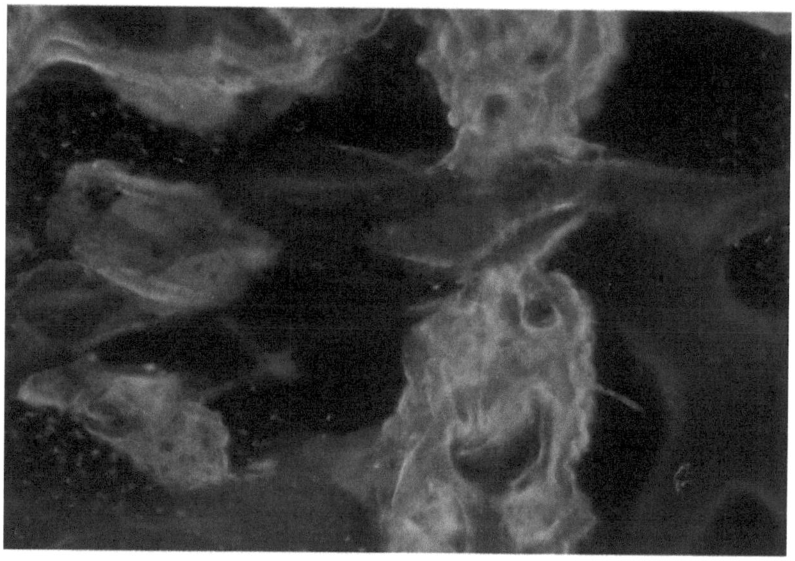

0,1 mm

Fig. 61. Gap healing with secondary remodelling coming from the cortex: In a few cases, osteons of the cortex have already started to cross the gap filled with lamellar bone, in a longitudinal direction (sheep 4213, group "compression with one plate")

Fig. 62. Microradiography of the osteotomy zone in sheep 15 (group "compression with two gauge plates"): A large intracortical resorption cavity reduces the weight bearing cross section of the bone

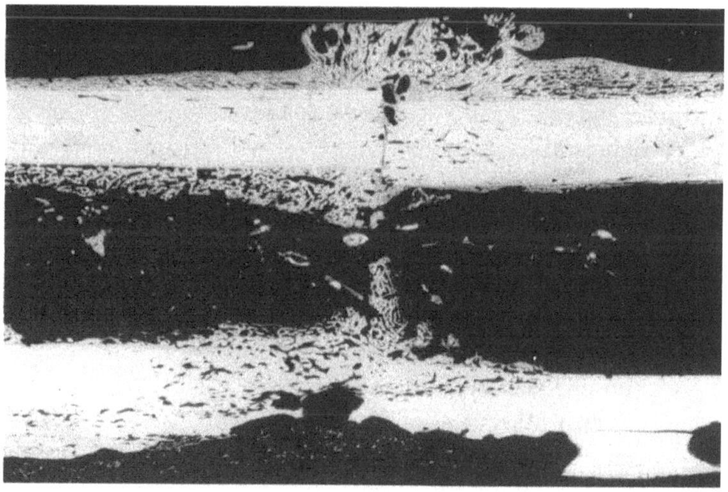

5 mm

The three remaining sheep of this group exhibited *extensive sequestration* in the osteotomy zone. Bony union seemed to be achieved by appositional callus only.

Sheep:

16, 739 Extensive callus bridge on one side and incomplete bridging on the opposite side with partly rounded ends.

878 Periosteal callus bridge complete in some areas; rounded edges of the fragment ends without bridging in other areas.

Group "compression with one plate": characteristics of *primary bone healing* were found in one sheep only.

Sheep: 4213 There was bony union by gap healing on the whole cortical circumference. Only few resorption zones or little callus were found.

In one sheep *no signs of bony union* between the fragment ends were found. There were however, no extensive resorptive changes.

Sheep: 23 A solid appositional callus secured the bony union of the fragments on one side, the callus bridge being incomplete on the opposite side with rounded edges and interposition of fibrous tissue.

In all other animals of this group extensive *sequestration* and solid, partly incomplete callus bridges were present.

Sheep:

279, 2665 On both sides of the circumference a solid callus bridge united the fragments.

1829 The callus bridge was complete only on one side of the cortex showing a gap in other areas of the circumference with rounded edges and interposition of fibrous tissue.

Group "no compression with one plate": signs of *primary bone healing* were found in two sheep.

Sheep:

1008, 847 On one side, gap healing was found, while extensive sequestration predominated[15] in the opposite cortex with formation of a callus which secured the bridging of this cortex.

In all other animals the osteotomy zone was *sequestrated* on both sides. Bony union was secured by *callus* only.

Sheep:

21, 24, 4212 On both sides of the circumference, union of the main fragments was secured by a complete callus bridge. This type of bony union occurred from the fifth to the eighth week.

785 Callus formation was very extensive but did not bridge the osteotomy completely on any of the cross sections.

[15] Therefore, these cases will not be classified as union of the primary type of bone healing.

4. Discussion

The treatment of infected osteosyntheses aims at two goals: union of the fracture and healing of the infection. These two goals often require contradictory actions, and the result of treatment of the infection by the removal of the implants compromises bone healing. The treatment of the fracture by leaving the implants *in situ*, or sometimes even performing a repeat osteosynthesis results in bony union but by paying the price of a long lasting infection which rarely ever heals before all implants can be removed [45]. Since both treatment regimes cure the infection in the long run, the treatment should primarily be directed towards the problem of bone repair. Just as in the healing process of the non-infected fracture, the biologic reaction of bone to mechanical influences may play an important role in the case of local infection [79]. For this reason we have concentrated in these experiments on the influence of the local infection on the biomechanics of the healing fracture.

The first question that arises is to what extent can the infectious changes and the mechanics of the experimental model be compared with the clinical situation. Remarkable similarity to human osteitis was found with regard to the morphological changes and sequential evolution of the *bone infection*, despite the species specificity reported in staphylococci [59]. Certain differences result from the fact that we infected the animals one week after surgery as opposed to immediate operative infection, mainly to avoid contamination and complications with asepsis in our operation theatres and in order to secure wound healing [32]. This difference was accepted because we were not so much concerned with imitating the evolution of the human disease in all details, but rather to study the effects of the infection, once it was started. We could achieve a bone infection lasting over the whole observation period of eight weeks in all animals: the bacteriologic control examinations repeatedly revealed the presence of bacteria, and on histologic examination, bacteria and round cells were found in close proximity to the osteotomy. Some methodological differences within the experiment as such (passages of bacterial cultures, see p. 14, and reinfection, see p. 23) could be another factor responsible for the disparity of the results, as could be the variability in the individual defence mechanism against infection.

With regard to the *mechanics* of our experimental model, a simple and easily reproducible transverse osteotomy represents a simplified fracture model. It results in a larger zone of contact between the main fragments when compared to a clinical fracture. It is however, more difficult to stabilise because of the smooth fracture planes. In earlier experiments [99, 84] we were able to show basically the same healing patterns in an osteotomy as are found in the fracture. Internal fixation of the osteotomised bone fragments in the animal experiment, where immediate unrestricted weight bearing takes place, cannot be performed with success using only a single "small" plate, as commonly done for repair of the fractured tibia in the human. We have therefore predominantly used double plates. Because this procedure (double-plating) became discredited in the clinical treatment of shaft fractures, we have studied an additional group of animals in which the osteotomy was stabilised with *a single*, although "large" plate.

A division into a group where interfragmentary compression was used and a group without such pressure effect seemed appropriate to create conditions similar to those with which the surgeons are often confronted: *i.e.* occasionally the surgeon deliberately avoids interfragmentary compression by the plate or is, in other cases, incapable of arriving at a resulting compression effect as shown by GALEAZZI [28]. The experimental model used imitates the spectrum of stability achieved in the clinical situation.

In the realm of diminished *stability,* the influence of local infection on fracture healing was tested by internal fixation without interfragmentary compression in addition to reduction of the cross section of the plate. A reduction of the thickness of the plate to 3 mm seemed to be an appropriate analogy to the data obtained by HUTZSCHENREUTER *et al.* [55], who regularly observed lack of osteotomy stability as indicated by resorption of the fragment ends and heavy callus formation in non-infected osteotomies stabilised with a 2.5 mm Syntacoben plate. We have had two fractures in the group without interfragmentary compression, occurring during the first postoperative week. They are thought to be the consequence of local overload of the bone in the area to which the implant is anchored [22]. In the absence of interfragmentary compression, the osteotomy plane does not participate in the force-transmission and the implant has to carry the full functional load. This may result in plate breakage or complete disruption of the implant, as can be seen in clinical cases, or it causes a fracture of the bone in the area to which the implant is fixed, as in the experimental animals described. Instability however, did not last long enough in the group "no compression with one plate" possibly because of the early and extensive callus formation under the conditions of the local infection. No difference between the group "no compression with one plate" and "compression with one plate" resulted with regard to bone healing as well as in the characteristics of the infectious disease. We shall therefore discuss the two groups together in the remaining part of this work. The osteotomies stabilised with two plates healed in spite of the infection, occasionally even in the manner of primary bone healing. The primary healing pattern in this group was found more frequently than in the groups with one plate only, a difference that proved to be statistically significant (four out of eight versus one out of eleven with $\chi^2 = 4.00$, $p < 0.05$).

The advantage of rigid fixation evidently outweighs the disadvantages which massive implants could have on the infectious disease. This leads to the conclusion that in the clinical treatment of infected fractures, optimal stability is the number one goal, regardless of the amount of implant material required to attain this aim. It would, however, not be acceptable in our view to conclude from these experiments that double plating should be recommended in the clinical management of bone infection. The stresses applied during the immediate postoperative phase in the experimental animal and the human are not comparable, as discussed on p. 63. Of uncertain significance is whether or not these results obtained with implants made of titanium can be applied easily to the results with implants made of other materials. Titanium has the advantage of high corrosion resistance [51, 103] and tissue tolerance [7]. The biomechanical disadvantages of double plating (stress protection [12]) can, however, only partly be avoided by the use of titanium, which is characterized by a comparatively low Young's modulus (11000 kp/mm^2).

On the basis of the results presented, the question arises as to whether or not further improvement in stability could possibly increase the number of primary bone healings. Such an improvement in stability could be achieved by arrangement of the two plates on opposite sides of the bones. This would, however, produce more soft tissue trauma. Also the evaluation of the effects of more extensive and longer lasting *in*stability on fracture healing and infection would be of great interest and worthy of further investigation.

The *in vivo measurements of interfragmentary compression* gave reliable information as to the stability of the osteosynthesis. The results are in accordance with those of the torque measure-

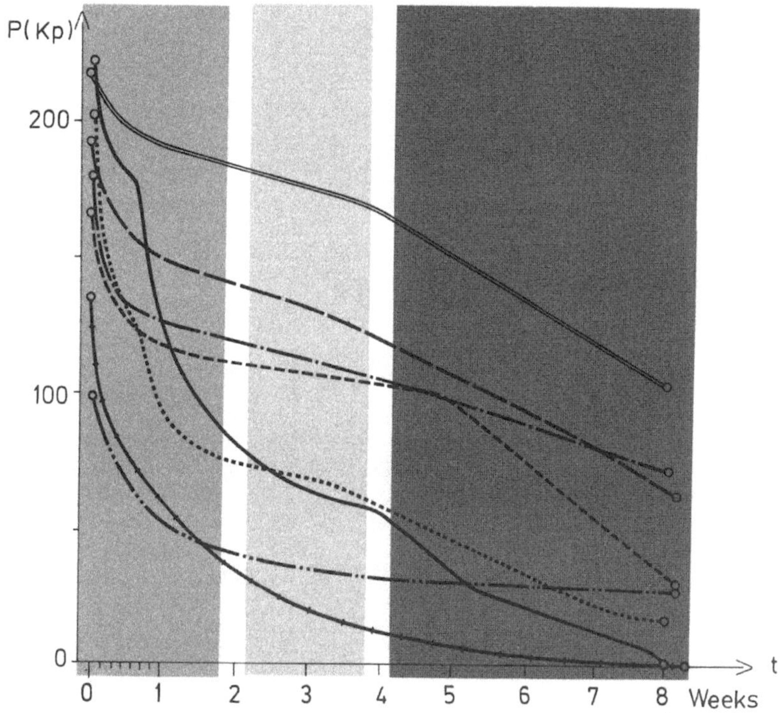

Fig. 63a. The three phases of the interfragmentary compression curve observed during the healing process of an infected bone: After an initial pressure drop a phase of slower reduction is seen. Following these two phases resembling the curves obtained under non-infected conditions, a third phase of accelerated pressure drop is often seen, starting after the fourth week and being specific for the infection

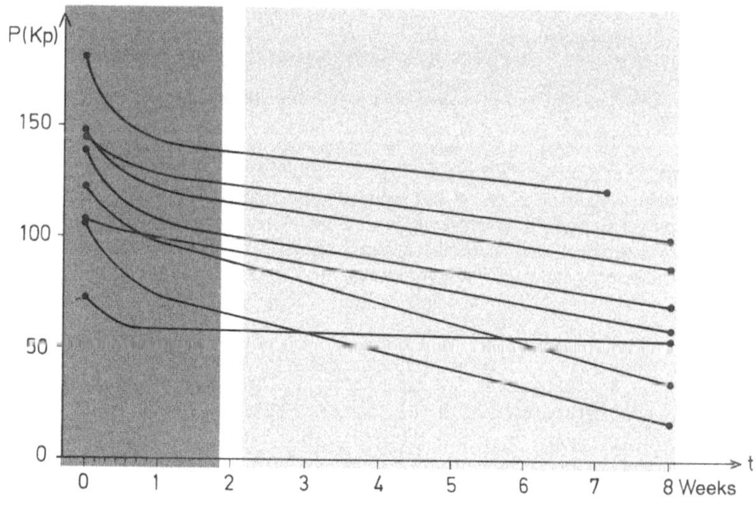

Fig. 63 b. The two phases of the pressure curve seen during the healing process of non-infected osteotomies: After an initial pressure loss a phase of slower further decrease is seen, which lasts until the end of the experiment. (From PERREN *et al.* [84])

ments and the data obtained with the electronic scale in respect to transmission of dynamic load to the gauge plates. The comparison of the changes in interfragmentary compression found in these infected osteotomies with the results obtained in analogous, non-infected experiments [84] shows a more rapid reduction in pressure within the first week (Fig. 63a and b) in the infected tissues. This could be due to the fact that the first measurement in the experiments presented was taken immediately after surgery, while in the non-infected studies mentioned, the first determination was only made following a lapse of a few hours after termination of the operative procedure. The two animals (sheep 821, 16) which showed a sudden second pressure drop on the fifth day had started off with high initial compression values. The sudden

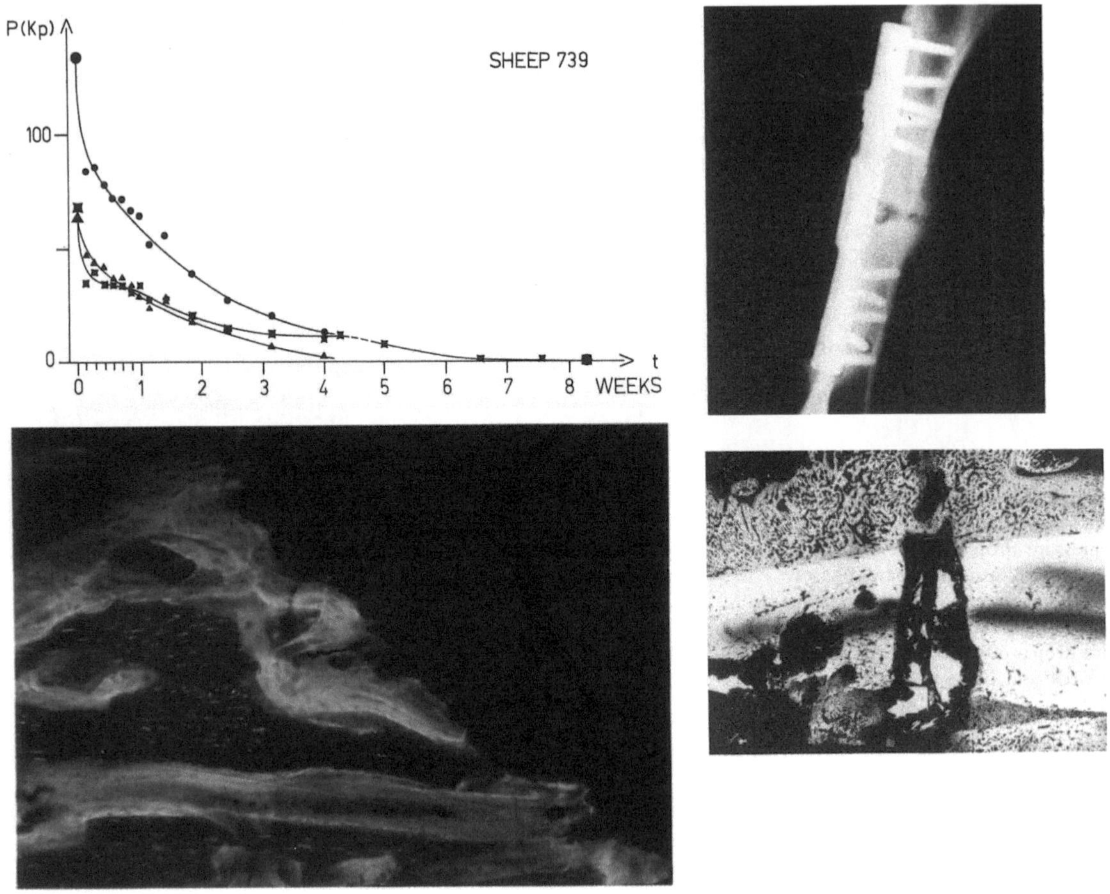

Fig. 64. Synopsis: Characteristics of the secondary healing pattern of infected bone. Biomechanical and biological aspects of the healing bone in sheep 739 (group "compression with two gauge plates"): The pressure curve shows an early collapse of the interfragmentary compression. After the fifth week, stability seems to be secured by the huge callus of cloudy structure. The osteotomy appears clearly widened with resorption fronts best seen on fluorescent microscopy. In radiographic and microradiographic pictures, extensive sequestra are prominent

drop was interpreted as local overload resulting from high *static* preload (220 kp and 200 kp, respectively, in the two sheep), associated with the additional *functional* charge at walking. Local zones of overload [89] can be seen in both cases on the microradiographic pictures (see p. 45, Fig. 37). In a third case (2287) with an initial interfragmentary compression of over 200 kp, no signs of local overload are found and the early pressure fall is not seen. The microradiography of this animal shows that a nearly ideal anatomical reposition with contact zones in the cortex of both sides of the longitudinal cut of the tibia had been achieved at surgery (optimal pressure distribution). The local overload found in the cortex of two animals however, points to the danger of excessive compression values. This is contrary to the recommendations recently published by Hess [40] who used up to 350 kp.

The pressure changes between the second and fourth weeks are similar in the infected and non-infected animals. It resembles the pressure curve found on intact bone [73] as well as in cortical bone transplants [56]. The results of the experiments cited suggested that Haversian remodelling is one of the important mechanisms responsible for the decrease in compression during the

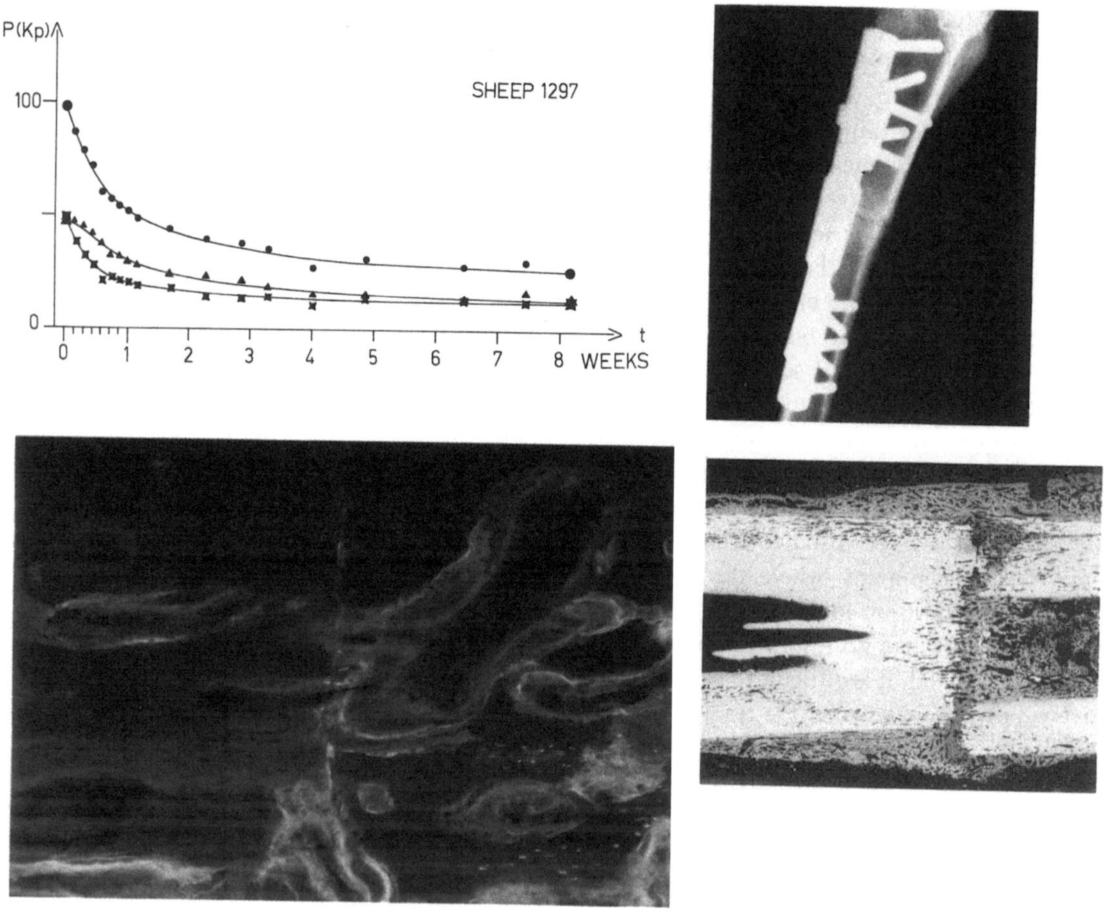

Fig. 65. Synopsis: Characteristics of primary bone healing in the presence of an infection. Biomechanical and biological aspects of the healing bone of sheep 1297 (group "compression with two gauge plates"): Interfragmentary compression remains active up to the end of the experiment, with no signs of accelerated terminal pressure drop. In comparison to the non-infected osteotomies however, a more rapid diminution is seen. On X-ray, beginning bony union with only slight callus formation. Fluorescent microscopy of the contact area shows osteons, which cross the osteotomy gap directly. Some single bone canals demonstrated a widened lumen. On microradiography, the contact zone and gap zone are seen in the process of healing. Little remodelling activity and "goccie di cera" filled with bone

second phase. Thereby, remodelling causes a replacement of prestretched bone by new bone which stands without tension. The direct relationship between bone remodelling and pressure reduction seems to be most conclusively demonstrated by HUTZSCHENREUTER'S [56] experiments (autogenous transplant: 59.5% pressure reduction and 48.6% remodelling rate; deproteinised allogen transplant: 39.2% pressure drop and 31.2% remodelling). In our experiments, the remodelling rate in the osteotomy zone examined is small. MATTER *et al.* [72], however, showed that very early after internal fixation, an active bone remodelling is to be expected near the screws.

In addition to the findings in non-infected osteotomies, our data suggest that processes other than the Haversian remodelling must be partly responsible for the reduction in compression. The rapid pressure drop which may be found under infectious conditions in the third phase goes along with extensive resorption (Fig. 64). On the other hand, those animals which showed a stable pressure plateau at medium or high pressure levels united in patterns resembling primary bone healing (Fig. 65). This shows very clearly that the pattern of bone healing is directly dependent on the stability of fixation, but it remains unclear why stability takes such a different course within the same group.

As a whole, compression measurements made on infected osteosyntheses have not shown any signs of pressure induced *bone necrosis* [58]; the resorptive processes have not been limited to the pressure zones. Within the area of osteotomy, localised zones of plastic bone deformation were found repeatedly and seemed to be caused by uneven surface pressure [89]. With regard to the sequestration of entire osteotomy zones, the question arises why the spheric erosions, which cause a sequestrum to break off, preferably occur at a given distance from the osteotomy. These same areas, where the bone is first eroded, demonstrate intensive remodelling activity in cases where no resorption of the osteotomy zone is found. It is difficult to answer conclusively the question whether the resorptive processes attack in the area of transition between well vascularised cortex and devascularised fragment ends. It is also striking that the osteotomy planes as such seem to be "selectively" exempted from the superficial resorptive processes. It is possible that an alteration of the fragment ends, as a consequence of the process of sawing at the time of osteotomy, could play a role, since in the presence of the dense vascular network found in the vicinity of the osteotomy, resorptive processes should really be expected to occur. Very infrequently sequestra do become revascularised [109]. This occurred only where the sequestra had been connected to the callus bridge which only later became separated. Our observations are in accordance with the assumption of Hicks [42] that sequestra—as a rule—are free from callus. However, they also show that such attachment of callus to a sequestrum is not impossible in principle.

In addition to the changes in interfragmentary compression, the *torque measurements* of the screws were a second parameter to evaluate the stability of implants. Torque (*M*) is directly related to the effective transverse compression (*N*) [5] and transverse compression to friction (*R*) between plate and bone surface [37]. It was, therefore, interesting to analyse the forces on the basis of the torque measurements which could still be transmitted at the end of the experiments in the longitudinal axis between plate and bone on the basis of friction. The correlation between axial force and torque can be calculated using the following formula [73]:

$$N=(M_x-M_0)\cdot K$$

N = force in direction of screw axis,
M_x = torque applied,
M_0 = torque required to overcome friction as long as no longitudinal force in the screw axis is present,
K = constant of Von Arx [5] = 7.2 cm^{-1}.

In technological fields, friction plays an important role in force transmission accomplished by joint connections. In our experiments friction is found on the contact planes between plate and bone surface and results from the compression force exerted by the screws [5]. The friction coefficient was found to be 0.38 [37]. The correlation between friction and axial force can be calculated using the following formula:

$$R=\mu\cdot N$$

R = maximum friction when plate is moved longitudinally on the bone surface,
μ = static friction coefficient of Hayes *et al.* [37] = 0.38.

With this formula the axial force necessary to move the plate on the bone was calculated using the following equation:

$$N=\frac{(L-4)+(A-2)}{2}\cdot K$$

$(L-4)$ represents the greater friction, with the added component between screw head and plate hole, while $(A-2)$ represents the smaller friction component between bone and screw. At implantation 3 cm·kp torque (M_0) [73] was required to overcome the screw-bone friction. Calculating the friction which was initially effective (*i.e.* at surgery) in the worst case (the most effective screw of the least-held plate) one comes up with a value of $(10-3)\cdot 7.2 = 50$ kp per screw on one side of the plate. Most often however, initial friction forces (interpreted as axial force) of $(\geqq 20-3)\cdot 7.2 \geqq 120$ kp were found. At the termination of the experiments, the friction values calculated were of such magnitude that they could account for the transmission of axial forces between bone and the implant of each animal with the exception of sheep 1297. In our opinion, this illustrates the important role friction forces play with regard to transmission of shear forces between plate and bone.

In addition to the examinations made to study the static forces (measurement of interfragmentary compression and torque), the effect of *dynamic* stress was studied by registration of the pressure changes with the animal walking. Considering the fact that micromotion is found as soon as the dynamic pressure load becomes larger than static preload [106, 85], it is of interest that in two sheep (739, 16) no static preload was found at the end of the experiment. Where this situation had existed for three weeks or longer (sheep 739), the implant had become loose. In the two sheep with pressure loss and loosening of the implant, the bacteriologic changes and clinical aspects of the infection did not differ before or after loosening of the implant, when compared with other animals.

The comparison of clinical *radiology, microradiography* and *histology* has shown, in all cases, a good correlation among these methods of evaluation with regard to the size of the fracture gap. The extent of callus was well recognised on X-ray in 18 out of 19 sheep. In 2 out of 14 cases sequestra were not apparent on the X-rays, and in 3 animals they were slightly underestimated. The diagnosis of osteolytic processes corresponded well, generally, when comparing the different diagnostic criteria; these changes were over- or underestimated on X-ray in only three cases each. The X-ray technique used for the explanted bone after removal of soft tissue, a method with which the clinician is not familiar, demonstrated the fracture lines with more contrast and could be interpreted as suggesting a lack of healing. However we would not go so far as GEISER [31], who, as late as 1963, said that "the radiologic control of callus formation had to be of only little benefit". We find in general a good correlation between X-ray changes and histology with regard to frequency, timing and quantity of the changes.

5. Summary and Conclusions

The results of the operative managment of fractures may be subject to question in the presence of infection. To study fracture healing in the presence of local infection, we performed transverse tibial osteotomies in sheep and stabilised them using different types of plate fixations. Thereafter, human-pathogenic staphylococci were injected locally and produced a chronic bone infection with fistulae, sequestrum formation, osteolysis and callus apposition similar to the condition in human osteitis. After eight weeks 18 out of 19 osteotomies showed patterns of bony union, even partly exhibiting the characteristics of primary bone healing. *In vivo* measurements of interfragmentary compression showed in most cases a different pattern when compared with the curve earlier described in non-infected osteotomies: a rapid pressure decrease is found between the fourth and the eighth week. In these cases resorption and sequestrum formation were extensive. The measurements of interfragmentary compression showed a good correlation between stability of the fixation and type of bone healing.

We have arrived at the following conclusions from the experiments presented:

1. The model presented qualifies for studying infectious changes and bone repair of an infected osteosynthesis.

2. Rigid fixation of the fragments offers favourable conditions for healing of the fracture. It is therefore advantageous to leave stabilising implant material *in situ* when an infection is present and furthermore to submit the patient to repeat osteosynthesis when an infected fracture has become unstable.

3. Primary bone healing is of great advantage where an infection is present, since it goes along with minimal sequestration.

4. The advantage of the stabilising effect of implants outweighs the disadvantages of a foreign body effect.

5. The appearance of callus after internal fixation and infection is not necessarily a sign of instability. On the contrary, the callus plays an important role in fracture healing in this condition.

Acknowledgments

We should like to thank many people who have contributed through their help and suggestions to this work:

P. Matter (M.D.), A. Rösli (M.D.) and D. Sunaric (M.D.) gave their competent medical advice.

We thank J. McDaniel (M.D.) and Miss P. Hall for the english translation of the text.

We are especially grateful to J. Schmid for his technical assistance during experimentation and bacteriologic examination; M. Bellasi for the photographic documentation; R. Damlund, E. Küng, and K. Nater for the histological work-up and P. Hall for performing the sheep anaesthesia. Additional important help was offered by U. Aeberhard, T. Geiser, M. Klebl, U. Matzner, R. Moor, E. Omerbegovič, B. Rahn (M.D.), and E. Rampoldi. E. Oberli helped to illustrate the text with his drawings.

Davos, July 31th, 1973

Literature

1. AEBERHARD, H.: Der Einfluß der Plattenüberbiegung auf die Torsionsstabilität der Osteosynthese. Bern: Med. Diss. (1973).
2. ALLGOEWER, M., PERREN, S., MATTER, P.: A new plate for internal fixation, the Dynamic Compression Plate (DCP). Injury **2**, 40 (1970).
3. ALLGOEWER, M.: Weichteilprobleme und Infektionsrisiko der Osteosynthese. Arch. klin. Chir. **329**, 1128 (1971).
4. ANDERSON, L. D.: Compression plate fixation and the effect of different types of internal fixation on fracture healing. J. Bone Jt Surg. **47-A**, 191 (1965).
5. VON ARX, C.: Schubübertragung durch Reibung bei Plattenosteosynthesen. Basel: Med. Diss. (1973).
6. BAGBY, G.W., JANES, J.M.: The effect of compression on the rate of fracture healing using a special plate. Amer. J. Surg. **95**, 761 (1958).
7. BECHTOL, C. O., FERGUSON, A. B., LAING, P. G.: Metals and engineering in bone and joint surgery. Baltimore: Williams & Wilkins 1959.
8. BEDACHT, R., FREY, K.-W., METZ, H., SCHAUER, A.: Vergleichende tierexperimentelle Untersuchungen mit autologen und heterologen Implantaten im Tibiaknochen beim Kaninchen. Ärztl. Forsch. **26**, 47 (1972).
9. BILLROTH, zit. nach LUNDSGAARD-HANSEN, P.: Antibiotica in der Chirurgie. Aktuelle Probleme in der Chirurgie, vol. **9**, p. 82 Bern/Stuttgart: Huber 1968.
10. BLAIR, J.E., WILLIAMS, R.E.O.: Phage typing of Staphylococci. Bull. Org. mond. Santé **24**, 771 (1961).
11. BOESENBERG, H.: Osteomyelitis, Erreger und Krankheitsbild. Hippokrates **38**, 460 (1967).
12. BRENNWALD, J., PERREN, S. M.: Bestimmung der Knochendehnung in vitro und in vivo nach Plattenosteosynthese. Arch. klin. Chir. Suppl. Chir. Forum **39** (1972).
13. BURKHARDT, R.: Farbatlas der klinischen Histopathologie von Knochenmark und Knochen. Berlin/Heidelberg/New York: Springer 1970.
14. BURRI, C.: Posttraumatische Osteitis. Bern/Stuttgart/Wien: Huber 1974.
15. CHARKES, N. D., SKLAROFF, D. M.: Early diagnosis of metastatic bone cancer by photoscanning with strontium^{85}. J. nucl. Med. **5**, 168 (1964).
16. CHARNLEY, J.: Compression arthrodesis. London: Livingstone 1953.
17. DANIS, R.: Théorie et pratique de l'ostéosynthèse. Paris: Masson 1947.
18. DECOULX, P.: L'infection opératoire en orthopédie. Les conditions de l'intervention. Rev. Chir. orthop. **55**, 194 (1969).
19. DEHNE, E., DEFFER, P. A., HALL, R. M., BROWN, P. W., JOHNSON, E. V.: The natural history of the fractured tibia. Surg. Clin. N. Amer. **41**, 1, 495 (1961).
20. DILMAGHANI, A., CLOSE, J. R., RHINELANDER, F. W.: A method for closed irrigation and suction therapy in deep wound infections. J. Bone Jt Surg. **51-A**, 323 (1969).
21. DOMBROWSKI, E. T., DUNN, A. W.: Treatment of osteomyelitis by debridement and closed wound irrigation-suction. Clin. Orthop. **43**, 215 (1965).
22. DWYER, N.: The protective influence of compression used in internal fixation on recently osteotomized rabbit tibiae. Injury **2**, 22 (1970).
23. EDWARDS, P.: The effect of crush injury to the skin on the healing fracture of the shaft of the tibia in dogs. Acta orthop. scand. **36**, 89 (1964).
24. ELLIS, H.: A study of some factors affecting prognosis following tibial shaft fractures. Oxford: Thesis. (1956).
25. FEISCHL, P.: Mischinfektion und bakteriologische Resistenzprobleme bei der posttraumatischen Osteomyelitis. In: HIERHOLZER, G., REHN, J.: Die posttraumatische Osteomyelitis, Stuttgart/New York: Schattauer 1970.
26. FLACH, K.: Die posttraumatische Osteomyelitis im Röntgenbild. In: Therapie der posttraumatischen Osteomyelitis. Schriftenreihe Unfallmedizinische Tagungen der Landesverbände der gewerblichen Berufsgenossenschaften **10**, 23 (1970).
27. FOGELBERG, E. V., ZITZMANN, E. K., STINCHFIELD, F. E.: Prophylactic penicillin on orthopaedic surgery. J. Bone Jt Surg. **52-A**, 95 (1970).
28. GALEAZZI, G.: Experimentelle Untersuchungen zur intraoperativen Druckveränderung bei der Plattenosteosynthese. Basel: Med. Diss. (1972).
29. GALLINARO, P., PERREN, S., CROVA, M., RAHN, B.: La osteosintesi con placca a compressione. In: ROASENDA, F., LORENZI, G. L.: Moderni orientamenti nelle osteosintesi delle fratture diafisarie. 54. Congr. SIOT, Roma (1969).
30. GALLINARO, P., RAHN, B. A., FILOGAMO, G.: The effect of compression in internal fixation of transverse osteotomies in rabbits. Europ. Surg. Res. **1**, 171 (1969).
31. GEISER, M.: Beiträge zur Biologie der Knochenbruchheilung. Stuttgart: Enke 1963.
32. GIERHAKE, F. W.: Postoperative Wundheilungsstörungen. Berlin/Heidelberg/New York: Springer 1970.
33. GREEN, M., NYHAN, W. L., and FOUSEK, M. D.: Acute hematogenous osteomyelitis. Pediatrics **17**, 368 (1956).
34. GRUNDMANN, G.: Experimentelle Untersuchungen zur Pathogenese der Osteomyelitis. Arch. klin. Chir. **277**, 117 (1953).

35. Hampton, O.P., Fitts, W.T. Jnr.: The open reduction of common fractures. New York/London: Grune and Stratton 1959.
36. Hayashi, I., Yanagibashi, H.: Effects of injuries on the development of myelitis; a study of experimental myelitis. (jap.). Orthop. Surg. **21**, 231 (1970).
37. Hayes, W.C., Perren, S.M.: Plate-bone friction in the compression fixation of fractures. Clin. Orthop. **89**, 236 (1972).
38. Hertel, E., Jani, L.: Probleme der Frakturheilung bei der Osteomyelitis. Beitr. Orthop. **15**, 2 (1958).
39. Hertel, E., Albrecht, R.: Die Dauerspüldrainage, Probleme und Erfahrungen bei der Behandlung sekundär-chronischer Osteomyelitiden. Z. Orthop. **104**, 260 (1968).
40. Hess, H.: Die Spannungskräfte der Druckplattenosteosynthese. In: Otte, P., Schlegel, K.F.: Bücherei des Orthopäden, vol. **9**, Stuttgart: Enke 1972.
41. Hicks, J.H.: The relationship between metal and infection. Proc. roy. Soc. Med. **50**, 842 (1957).
42. Hicks, J.H.: Non-union of fractures. Lancet **1963 I**, 86.
43. Hicks, J.H.: Amputation in fractures of the tibia. J. Bone Jt Surg. **46-B**, 388 (1964).
44. Hicks, J.H.: The treatment of chronic sepsis in fractures. J. Bone Jt Surg. **47-B**, 584 (1965).
45. Hicks, J.H.: Sepsis in fractures. In: London, P.S.: Modern trends in accident surgery and medicine 2. London: Butterworth 1970.
46. Hierholzer, G., Knothe, H., Rehn, J., Koch, F.: Fusidinsäure-Konzentrationen in chronisch entzündlichem Gewebe. Arzneimittelforsch. **16**, 1549 (1966).
47. Hierholzer, G., Rehn, J.: Zur Indikation einer zusätzlichen antibiotischen Therapie bei der chronischen Knocheninfektion. Tagung der mittelrheinischen Chirurgenvereinigung, Homburg (1966).
48. Hierholzer, G., Rehn, J., Koch, F., Gatos, M.: Untersuchungen zur chronischen Osteomyelitis, 1. Beeinflussung des Keimwachstums in chronisch entzündetem Knochengewebe durch Antibiotika. Bruns Beitr. klin. Chir. **215**, 376 (1967).
49. Hierholzer, G.: Klinisch-experimentelle Untersuchungen zur Therapie der chron. Osteomyelitis mit einem Steroidantibioticum. In: Therapie der posttraumatischen Osteomyelitis. Schriftenreihe Unfallmedizinische Tagungen der Landesverbände der gewerblichen Berufsgenossenschaften, **10**, 81 (1970).
50. Hierholzer, G., Rehn, J.: Die posttraumatische Osteomyelitis. Stuttgart/New York: Schattauer 1970.
51. Hoar, T.P., Mears, D.: Corrosion-resistant alloys in chloride solutions: materials for surgical implants. Proc. roy. Soc. A. **239**, 486 (1966).
52. Holderman, W.D.: Results following conservative treatment of fractures of the tibial shaft. Amer. J. Surg. **98**, 593 (1959).
53. Huener, H., Schicker, H., Dollmann, R.: Möglichkeiten, Grenzen und Gefahren der modernen Therapie der akuten haematogenen Osteomyelitis. Chirurg **33**, 405 (1962).
54. Hunter, J.: Lectures on the principles of surgery from the works of John Hunter. Ed. by James F. Palmer, London: Longman 1835.
55. Hutzschenreuter, P., Perren, S.M., Steinemann, S., Geret, V., Klebl, M.: Some effects of rigidity of internal fixation on the healing pattern of osteotomies. Injury **1**, 77 (1969).
56. Hutzschenreuter, P.: Beschleunigte Einheilung von allogenen Knochentransplantaten durch Praesensibilisierung des Empfängers und stabile Osteosynthese. Arch. klin. Chir. **331**, 321 (1972).
57. Jantke, W., Wenta, H.: Chemotherapeutische Frühbehandlung und Prophylaxe in der Unfallchirurgie. Münch. med. Wschr. **12**, 662 (1969).
58. Jores, L.: Experimentelle Untersuchungen über die Einwirkung mechanischen Druckes auf den Knochen. Beitr. path. Anat. **66**, 433 (1920).
59. Israel, L.: Staphylococci in animals: differentiation and relationship to human Staphylococcosis In: Cohen, J.O.: The Staphylococci, Library of Congress Cataloging, in Publication Data. New York/London/Sydney/Toronto: Wiley 1972.
60. Kallenberger, A., Roth, W., Ledermann, M.: Experimentelle bakteriologische Untersuchungen zur Wahl des Spülmittels für die antibakterielle Spüldrainage. In: Hierholzer, G., Rehn, J.: Die posttraumatische Osteomyelitis, Stuttgart/New York: Schattauer 1970.
61. Key, J.A.: Positive pressure in arthrodesis for tuberculosis of the knee joint. Sth med. J. **25**, 909 (1932).
62. Kocher, T.: Zur Ätiologie der akuten Entzündung. Arch. klin. Chir. **23**, 101 (1878).
63. Kuner, E., Houschyar, K., Weyand, F.: Das Osteomyelitisproblem im Wandel der Prophylaxe und Therapie. Bruns Beitr. klin. Chir. **219**, 46 (1971).
64. Lane, W.A.: zitiert nach Hicks [41].
65. Lennert, K.: Grundprobleme der Osteomyelitis. Verh. dtsch. orthop. Ges. Z. Orthop. Suppl. **100**, 27 (1965).
66. Lexer, E.: Die freien Transplantationen. In: Neue deutsche Chirurgie, vol. **26**, Stuttgart: Enke 1924.
67. Linzenmeier, G., Schaefer, P., Volk, H., Gatos, M.: Bestimmung der Konzentration von Lincomycin in chronisch entzündetem Knochen- und Weichteilgewebe des Menschen. Arzneimittelforsch. **18**, 204 (1968).
68. Linzenmeier, G.: Bakteriologische Probleme der posttraumatischen Osteomyelitis. In: Hierholzer, G., Rehn, J.: Die posttraumatische Osteomyelitis, Stuttgart/New York: Schattauer 1970.
69. Lister, J.: On a new method of treating compound fracture, abscess etc. Lancet **1867 I**, 326.
70. Lubegina, Z.: Bone tissue regeneration under conditions of chronic infection, (Rus.) Ortop. travm. Protez **27**, 17 (1966).
71. Luedeke, H., Schweiberer, L.: Entzündliche Erkrankungen des Knochens und der Gelenke. Chirurg **41**, 204 (1970).
72. Matter, P., Brennwald, J., Rueter, A., Perren, S.M.: Die knöcherne Heilung von Schraubenlöchern nach Metallentfernung. Z. Orthop. **110**, 920 (1972).
73. Matter, P.: Knochenumbau bei der Druckplattenosteosynthese; Habilitationsschrift (1973).
74. Matter, P., Rittmann, W.W.: In Bearbeitung.
75. Mecseki, L., Kosik, G., Herics, I.: Die primäre Osteosynthese bei offenen Unterschenkelbrüchen. Beitr. Orthop. **16**, 201 (1969).
76. Mittelmeier, H.: Zur Entstehung und Bedeutung der exogenen Osteomyelitis. In: Hierholzer, G., Rehn, J.: Die posttraumatische Osteomyelitis, Stuttgart/New York: Schattauer 1970.
77. Moe, J.H.: Prevention and treatment of infections in bone. J. Lancet **79**, 2 (1959).

78. MÜLLER, H. J.: Äußere Fixation bei posttraumatischer Osteomyelitis, Indikation, Technik, Ergebnisse, Weiterversorgung. In: Therapie der posttraumatischen Osteomyelitis. Schriftenreihe Unfallmedizinische Tagungen der Landesverbände der gewerblichen Berufsgenossenschaften, **10**, 81 (1970).
79. MÜLLER, M. E., ALLGÖWER, M., WILLENEGGER, H.: Manual der Osteosynthese (AO-Technik). Berlin/Heidelberg/New York: Springer 1969.
80. NORDEN, C. W.: Experimental osteomyelitis. I. A description of the model. J. infect. Dis. **122**, 410 (1970).
81. NORDEN, C. W.: Experimental Osteomyelitis. II. Therapeutic trials and measurement of antibiotic levels in bone. J. infect Dis. **124**, 565 (1971).
82. PAPASTAVROU, N., ECKE, H.: Zur Leistungsfähigkeit der antibakteriellen Spüldrainage. Bruns Beitr. klin. Chir. **218**, 255 (1970).
83. PERREN, S. M., HUGGLER, A., RUSSENBERGER, M., STRAUMANN, F., MÜLLER, M. E., ALLGÖWER, M.: A method of measuring the change in compression applied to living cortical bone. Acta orthop. scand. Suppl. **125**, 7 (1969).
84. PERREN, S. M., RUSSENBERGER, M., STEINEMANN, S., MÜLLER, M. E., ALLGÖWER, M.: A dynamic compression plate. Acta orthop. scand. Suppl. **125**, 29 (1969).
85. PERREN, S. M., GANZ, R., RÜTER, A.: Mechanical induction of bone resorption. 4th Int. Osteological Symp., Prag 1972.
86. POPKIROV, S.: Die Behandlung der haematogenen und traumatischen Osteomyelitis. Berlin: VEB, Volk und Gesundheit 1971.
87. RAHN, B. A., PERREN, S. M.: Calcein blue as a fluorescent label in bone. Experientia **26**, 519 (1970).
88. RAHN, B.A., PERREN, S.M.: Xylenol orange, a fluorochrome useful in polychrome sequential labeling of calcifying tissues. Stain Technol. **46**, 125 (1971).
89. RAHN, B.A., GALLINARO, P., SCHENK, R.K., BALTENSPERGER, A., PERREN, S.M.: Compression interfragmentaire et surcharge locale de l'os. In: BOITZY'S, A.: Périarthrite de l'épaule. Berne/Stuttgart/Vienne: Huber 1972.
90. RAHN, B. A., PERREN, S. M.: Alizarinkomplexon-Fluorochrom zur Markierung von Knochen- und Dentinanbau. Experientia **28**, 180 (1972).
91. REHN, J.: Markphlegmonen nach Marknagelungen. In: HIERHOLZER, G., REHN, J.: Die posttraumatische Osteomyelitis. Stuttgart/New York: Schattauer 1970.
92. REYNOLDS, F. C., ZAEPFEL, F.: Management of chronic osteomyelitis secondary to compound fractures. J. Bone Jt Surg. **30-A**, 331 (1948).
93. RHINELANDER, F. W., BARAGRY, R. A.: Microangiography in bone healing. I. Undisplaced closed fractures. J. Bone Jt Surg. **44-A**, 1273 (1962).
94. RITTMANN, W. W., GRUBER, U. F.: Antibiotica-Prophylaxe in der Chirurgie. Méd. Hyg. **27**, 786 (1969).
95. RITTMANN, W. W., PUSTERLA, C., MATTER, P.: Früh- und Spätinfektionen bei offenen Frakturen. Helv. chir. Acta **36**, 537 (1969).
96. ROWE, C. R., SAKELLARIDES, H. T.: Recent advances in treatment of osteomyelitis following fractures of the long bones. Surg. Clin. N. Amer. **41**, 1593 (1961).
97. ROWLING, D. E.: Experience in the management of chronic osteomyelitis. 5th int. Congr. Chemotherapy, Wien 1967.
98. SCHEMAN, L., LEWIN, P., SIDEMAN, S., JANOTA, M.: Experimental osteomyelitis. Amer. J. Surg. **60**, 371 (1943).
99. SCHENK, R., WILLENEGGER, H.: Zum histologischen Bild der sogenannten Primärheilung der Knochenkompakta nach experimentellen Osteotomien am Hund. Experientia **19**, 593 (1963).
100. SCHENK, R. K.: Zur histologischen Verarbeitung von unentkalktem Knochen. Acta anat. **60**, 3 (1965).
101. SCOTT, J. C.: In: CLARK, J. M.: Modern trends in orthopaedics, 3. London: Butterworths 1962.
102. SIMONIS, G., BRÜHL, P.: Erregermosaik und aktuelle Resistenzsituation bei Verlaufsbeobachtungen der posttraumatischen Osteomyelitis. In: HIERHOLZER, G., REHN, J.: Die posttraumatische Osteomyelitis. Stuttgart/New York: Schattauer 1970.
103. STEINEMANN, S.: persönl. Mitt.
104. STEVENS, D. B.: Postoperative orthopaedic infections. A study of etiological mechanisms. J. Bone Jt Surg. **48-A**, 96 (1964).
105. TSCHERNE, H.: Operative Frakturbehandlung. Arch. klin. Chir. **324**, 348 (1969).
106. WAGNER, H.: Die Einbettung von Metallschrauben im Knochen und die Heilungsvorgänge des Knochengewebes unter dem Einfluß der stabilen Osteosynthese. Arch. klin. Chir. **305**, 28 (1963).
107. WALDVOGEL, F.A., MEDOFF, G., SWARTZ, M.N.: Osteomyelitis, clinical features, therapeutic considerations and unusual aspects. Springfield: Thomas 1971.
108. WATSON-JONES, R.: zit. in HICKS, J. H. [44].
109. WILLENEGGER, H., ROTH, W.: Die antibakterielle Spüldrainage als Behandlungsprinzip bei chirurgischen Infektionen. Dtsch. med. Wschr. **30**, 1485 (1962).
110. WILLENEGGER, H.: Behandlung von Infektionen des oberen Sprunggelenkes nach offenen Brüchen und nach operativer Behandlung geschlossener Brüche. H. Unfallhlk. **92**, 71 (1967).

Subject-Index

abscess 15, 21, 23, 25, 26, 50
alizarin complexone 17, 52
amputation 1
anaesthesia 7
antibiotics 2, 20
autopsy 19, 21, 24, 26

bacteria 1, 4, 13, 14, 20, 21, 22, 23, 24, 25, 26, 27, 63
—, counts 14, 15, 20
bacteriologic examination 14, 15, 19, 20, 21, 22, 23, 24, 25, 26, 27, 63
bacteriophages s. phage type
biomechanics 2, 3, 63
blood agar plates 14, 15, 22, 25, 27
bone
—, deposition 16, 54, 56, 59
—, healing 2, 20, 40, 55, 57, 63, 64, 69
—, healing primary 2, 40, 43, 49, 55, 60, 61, 62, 64, 67
—, healing secondary 2, 40, 42, 49, 50, 66
—, lamellar 52, 55, 57, 58, 60
—, necrosis 68
—, remodelling s. Haversian remodelling
—, transplant 67
bony union 20, 40, 49, 57, 58, 62
bridge amplifier 11, 12, 13, 27

calcein blue 17, 52
calcein green 17, 52
calibration 12, 26
callus 2, 16, 21, 40, 41, 42, 49, 50, 51, 52, 55, 57, 58, 60, 62, 64, 68, 69
carrier frequency amplifier s. bridge amplifier
chemoprophylaxis 2
Cl. Welchii 19
compression s. interfragmentary compression
—, transverse 12, 68
contact healing 55, 57, 58, 59, 66, 67
corrosion resistance 5, 64
C. pyogenes 24, 25, 26

decalcification 18
deformation, elastic 11, 29
—, plastic 11, 29
diastasis 4, 5, 9, 10, 35, 64
dipht. rods 25, 26
double plating 5, 6, 8, 63, 64
dynamic compression plate 5, 6
dynamometer 12

E. coli 1, 19, 24, 25, 26
encephalitis 20, 25
erosion s. resorption
experimental osteitis 1, 2, 3, 63
explantation 12, 16, 17
external fixation device 2

Faxitron 16, 40, 41, 44, 45, 46, 47, 48, 49, 69
fibrous bone 52, 57
—, tissue 62
fistula 14, 15, 20, 21, 23, 24, 26
fluorochromes 17, 52, 54
force transmission 13, 36, 37, 38, 39, 64, 68
—, transposition 33, 65
foreign body effect 2, 63, 64
fracture 19, 20, 63, 64
—, gap 4, 9, 10, 16, 35, 40, 41, 42, 44, 69
friction 12, 13, 68
fungus infection 25

Gallamine-Giemsa 18
gap healing 57, 58, 60, 61, 62, 67
gauge plate 4, 6, 8, 10, 11, 26, 27, 28, 29, 30, 31, 36, 37, 38, 39
germs s. bacteria
Goccie di cera 54, 55, 56, 58, 67
granulation tissue 2, 26

Haemalaune-eosin 18
Haversian canal 2
—, remodelling 16, 50, 52, 54, 56, 57, 58, 61, 66, 67, 68
healing s. bone healing
histology 1, 17, 49, 69

implant 2, 4, 5, 7, 8, 9, 10, 28, 29, 30, 31
—, chemical properties 5
—, loosening 36
—, mechanical properties 5
—, removal 2, 63
Indian ink 16, 50, 53
infection 13, 14, 15, 63
—, complication 19, 20, 26
—, frequency 1
—, healing 63
—, risk 1
inoculum 14, 15
instability 4, 5, 9, 64, 69
instruments 6
insulation 11, 12, 30
interfragmentary compression 2, 4, 5, 7, 8, 9, 10, 11, 26, 36, 37, 38, 39, 63, 64, 65, 66
—, changes 4, 27, 30, 31, 32, 33, 34, 35, 36
—, measurement 4, 10, 11, 13, 26, 27, 28, 29, 30, 31, 32, 33, 34, 35, 36, 64, 65, 66
internal fixation 7, 8, 9, 10

labelling 16, 17, 51, 52, 54, 55, 56, 58, 59, 60, 61
leucocytes 2, 53, 56, 58
load-strain diagram 12
loading force 13, 36, 37, 38, 39, 64, 69
lyophilisate 4, 14

McConkey plate 15
mechanics 3
Megohm-meter 12
methods 4, 7
methyl methacrylate 16, 17, 18
mice passage 14, 15
microangiography 16, 50, 51, 53, 60
microfractures 68
micromotion 69
Micropaque 16, 50
microradiography 16, 18, 41, 44, 45, 46, 47, 48, 49, 50, 52, 53, 54, 55, 56, 57, 61, 69
microtome 17, 18
mixed infection 1, 20, 23, 24, 25, 26
monoinfection 23, 25

neisseria sp. 21, 23

operation 7, 8, 9, 10
osteoblast 2, 54
osteocyte 2, 56
osteolysis s. resorption
osteon 56, 58, 60, 61, 67
osteotomy 7, 17, 54, 55, 57, 59, 60, 63, 68
overload 66

pathogenesis 3
phage type 4, 14, 15, 21, 23, 24, 25, 26
plate 4, 5, 7, 8, 9, 10, 28, 29, 30, 31
platform, electronic 13, 36, 37, 38, 39
plugging 60
pneumococci 21, 23
pre-tension 6, 8, 9
proteus sp. 1
pseudarthrosis 2
pseudomonas sp. 1

radiography 1, 16, 40, 41, 42, 43, 44, 45, 46, 47, 48, 49, 69
remodelling s. Haversian remodelling
repeat osteosynthesis 63
revaccination 15, 20, 23, 24, 25
resorption 2, 16, 40, 41, 49, 50, 52, 53, 54, 55, 56, 57, 58, 59, 60, 61, 62, 64, 66, 67, 68, 69

saw cut 16, 17, 18
sclerosis 1, 16, 40, 41
screws 5, 6, 12, 68
screw hole 5, 6, 68
sequential labelling s. labelling
sequestrum 1, 16, 40, 41, 42, 49, 53, 54, 55, 57, 60, 62, 66, 68, 69
sheep 4
stability 2, 5, 8, 63, 64, 67, 68
staphylococcus
—, aureus 1, 4, 13, 14, 15, 19, 20, 21, 22, 23, 24, 25, 26, 27, 63
—, epidermidis 1, 21, 23, 24, 25, 26
streptococci 1, 21, 23, 24
stress protection 5, 64
superinfection 1, 23, 25
Syntacoben 64

temperature effect 11, 26, 27, 28
test rig 11, 12
therapy 2, 63
tissue tolerance 5, 64
titanium 4, 5, 64
torque 12, 35, 64, 68
—, of extraction 12, 36
—, of loosening 13, 35, 36

vascularity 2, 50, 51, 53, 57, 58, 60, 68
virulence 14
Volkmann's canal 2

weight bearing 7, 13, 20, 21, 36, 38, 39, 63
Wheatstone bridge 11
wire 8, 11, 12, 30
—, break 12, 30, 37, 38, 39
wound healing 20

xylenol orange 17, 52

M. E. Müller, M. Allgöwer,
H. Willenegger

Manual of Internal Fixation

Technique Recommended by the AO-Group (Swiss Association for the Study of Internal Fixation: ASIF). In collaboration with W. Bandi, H. R. Bloch, A. Mumenthaler, R. Schneider, B. G. Weber, S. Weller. Translated by J. Schatzker
306 figures (683 separate illustrations). IX, 297 pages. 1970
ISBN 3-540-05219-4 Cloth DM 174,–
ISBN 0-387-05219-4 (North America)
Cloth US $50.10

M. E. Müller, M. Allgöwer,
H. Willenegger

Technique of Internal Fixation of Fractures

With contributions by W. Bandi, H. R. Bloch, A. Mumenthaler, R. Schneider, S. Steinemann, F. Straumann, B. G. Weber. Revised for the English edition by G. Segmüller
244 figures. XII, 272 pages. 1965
ISBN 3-540-03374-2 Cloth DM 98,–
ISBN 0-387-03374-2 (North America)
Cloth US $29.80

The Dynamic Compression Plate (DCP)

By M. Allgöwer, P. Matter, S. M. Perren, T. Rüedi
26 figures. IV, 45 pages. 1973
ISBN 3-540-06466-4 DM 18,–
ISBN 0-387-06466-4 (North America)
US $9.90

Orthopedics

Compiled and edited by R. M. Hall
356 illustrations by T. Bloodhart
XIV, 509 pages. 1972
(Air Instrument Surgery, Vol. 2)
ISBN 3-540-05809-5 Cloth DM 140,–
ISBN 0-387-05809-5 (North America)
Cloth US $53.90
Distribution rights for Japan:
Nankodo Co. Ltd., Tokyo

M. Watanabe, S. Takeda, H. Ikeuchi

Atlas of Arthroscopy

Entirely revised second edition
134 figures in color. IX, 176 pages. 1970
ISBN 3-540-05268-2 Cloth DM 102,–
ISBN 0-387-05268-2 (North America)
Cloth US $34.90
Published by Igaku Shoin Ltd., Tokyo
Sole distribution rights for the USA, Canada, and Europe (including the United Kingdom): Springer-Verlag

---

Prices are subject to change without notice

Springer-Verlag
Berlin Heidelberg New York
München Johannesburg London
Madrid New Delhi Paris Rio de Janeiro
Sydney Tokyo Utrecht Wien

MIX
Papier aus verantwortungsvollen Quellen
Paper from responsible sources
FSC® C105338

If you have any concerns about our products,
you can contact us on
ProductSafety@springernature.com

In case Publisher is established outside the EU,
the EU authorized representative is:
Springer Nature Customer Service Center GmbH
Europaplatz 3, 69115 Heidelberg, Germany

Printed by Libri Plureos GmbH
in Hamburg, Germany